SAFE
Sexual Healing

A Guidebook for Healers and Clients

Sunyata Satchitananda

BALBOA.
PRESS
A DIVISION OF HAY HOUSE

Balboa Press books may be ordered through booksellers or by contacting:

Balboa Press
A Division of Hay House
1663 Liberty Drive
Bloomington, IN 47403
www.balboapress.com
1 (877) 407-4847

Print information available on the last page.

ISBN: 978-1-9822-3441-6 (sc)
ISBN: 978-1-9822-3442-3 (e)

Balboa Press rev. date: 09/06/2019

Contents

Preface

I've been an ordained minister and spiritual counselor since 1980, trained in helping couples resolve their relationship problems and deal with the issues that affect their spirituality. After my divorce in 2000 I began to study neo-Tantra and the subtle energy system of the body. In 2007 I became a Certified Tantric Healer (sexual healer) and have worked with 100s of clients who have been: psychotherapists, medical practitioners, alternative healers, shamans, sex coaches, sexual healers, and men and women of many other professions. My clients have been mostly cis-gendered women and men, and gay men.

This guidebook came about due to a "perfect storm" of reported complaints about client abuse during sessions with sexual healers— in addition to reported abuse by spiritual leaders, yoga teachers, life coaches, alternative healers, and energy workers. After reading comments in a sexual healing support Yahoo Group email thread which exposed abusive/assaultive treatment some women experienced with male sexual healers, I had a conversation with a fellow sexual healer who told me that several women had shared with him their experiences of being assaulted by male sexual healers during healing sessions.

Also during this time, a female colleague shared with me her experiences with other sexual healers and in sexual healing workshops which crossed consent boundaries and made her feel unsafe. In addition to all of this, I read comments on social media from women who were complaining about men who presented themselves as spiritual leaders or healers but who took advantage of a woman's vulnerability and acted inappropriately.

The impact of all these reports emphasized to me the extraordinary vulnerabilities that clients face and for the need of ethical integrity and harmlessness in all client-healer interactions if real healing is to have an opportunity. These sexual assault experiences represent what can happen when the shadow side of sexual healing is not addressed and prepared for with education and implementation of safer healing practices.

Thankfully, transgressions like what has been reported are not the experience for the majority of sexual healing clients. However, my reverence and compassion for women and my desire for men to be part of the solution and not the problem inspired me to contribute to this conversation what I feel are fundamental principles and guidelines to providing safe sexual healing. I'm not saying that female sexual healers don't also transgress with clients—safe sexual healing practices apply equally to them. However, from what I've been made aware of, it seems the vast majority of complaints are against male healers, teachers, and leaders in the Tantra/sexual healing, yoga, consciousness, and alternative healing communities.

What I heard directly from clients, colleagues, and saw being expressed concerning sexual healers from their clients, made me realize that there was a gap in awareness and understanding about the potential for harm; and a need for sound guidance on basic, essential principles of behavior to help put an end to harming survivors of sexual abuse or assault who are only seeking healing.

This guidebook is an opportunity to supply some needed insight on a subject about which not a lot is generally known—to help survivors seeking relief to be more aware and informed about sexual healing. And, it's an opportunity to help potential clients know what questions to ask a prospective sexual healer; and to know what to expect in a sexual healing session.

In addition, this guidebook is an opportunity to help sexual healers further appreciate their solemn responsibility in safely stewarding sexual healing sessions—to know what is important to be aware of and include in a session and to know what's important to do to avoid creating injury or harm to their clients.

To sexual healers:

Bless you, for taking on this very challenging and sensitive, intimate healing modality—and in shouldering the tremendous responsibility for the safety and wellbeing of your client. In this guidebook, I present some best practices while pointing out some of the dangers and vulnerabilities associated with this vital healing work.

The vast majority of you have integrity and the highest regard for your client. My hope is that this guidebook will help you sustain an awareness that promotes safe sexual healing practices for both your clients and yourself so that no harm is created.

To sexual trauma survivors seeking relief and considering working with a sexual healer:

Some of what you read in this guidebook might push your buttons and trigger your fears about getting help with healing from sexual abuse. The cited examples of misconduct or bad practices are meant to inform and forewarn you so you can make sound decisions in choosing a sexual healer who will be competent and responsible in aiding you in achieving your goal of healing and returning to wholeness.

You might not be ready to work with a sexual healer, and should instead work with a counselor or therapist until you feel ready for sexual healing. This guidebook presents several questions for you to consider which will help you determine if you are ready for sexual healing.

If a sexual healer follows the recommendations in this guidebook you can have confidence that they are someone that respects your safety and will act with integrity to safely steward your healing journey. How can you know? Ask the sexual healer if they have read this guidebook or received other training in sexual healing ethics. Training may be an indicator of competency but doesn't guarantee ethical behavior—so try to get referrals and meet with prospective healers prior to receiving any treatments.

Safe Sexual Healing

Just reading this guidebook won't certify anyone to be a Safe Sexual Healer. To be a safe sexual healer, the advice suggested herein must be put into practice, along with obtaining appropriate training that includes finding a mentor to receive feedback on implementing ethical sexual healing practices.

Sincere and conscientious sexual healers who have their client's welfare as their top priority deserve respect and appreciation for their sacred service in behalf of humanity's healing. My hope is that this guidebook spreads awareness and fosters discussion about the sensitive and vulnerable exposure to harm that a client faces when seeking their sexual healing.

My intent is to help healers from many methods and backgrounds, as well as help an uninformed public learn about safe sexual healing—and to strongly support a client's right to safe and competent healing services.

May this guidebook be included wherever ethics in sexual healing is the topic of discussion and be part of promoting a broader and deeper insight into this complex and much-needed healing modality.

—Sunyata Satchitananda

Introduction

Safety

For many people, *sexual healing* is a controversial and wildly *out there* alternative healing therapy which they know almost nothing about. That unfamiliarity about a deeply intimate subject, combined with the sensitive and vulnerable condition of those who have experienced sexual abuse or assault creates a lot of fear and trepidation. So, it's a worthwhile question to ask "Is it possible for someone to receive sexual healing—safely?"

There can be no 100% guarantee that no harm will occur as a result of sexual healing treatments—but that is also true of other commonly accepted medical or therapeutic treatments. What we can do, and what this book is dedicated to, is to make the likelihood of harm as small as possible. In this book, we will be looking at many of the ways that a client's safety should be considered and how safer healing policies and practices can be implemented.

Healing

A simple definition of healing is: *a positive transformation that provides relief from symptoms of dis-ease.* Sexual healing includes positive transformational shifts which profoundly impact and elevate a client's sense of self and wellbeing. And, sexual healing can also include less profound but still significant shifts that relieve less severe symptoms.

Experiencing *Healing* doesn't necessarily mean that a trauma survivor no longer remembers what happened to them. Hopefully, healing will mean that they think about the abuse less often and are not plagued by oppressive inner-narratives. It is a healing victory when a survivor is no longer emotionally thrown off, overwhelmed, fragmented, or compelled by their trauma or its triggers which would have previously overtaken them.

Ultimately healing is about positive transformation—and that is what I want to protect, and promote with this book. By collecting and presenting the information in this guidebook, my goal is to support safe, and positive transformation for people seeking help with healing from sexual and emotional trauma.

Healing can occur in unexpected settings and in unanticipated ways. In the world of sexual healing, there is a broad spectrum of activities and circumstances where it can be applied. There are counselors, coaches, therapists, and alternative healers who help people heal sexual trauma and improve their sex life. In addition, the growing worldwide interest in Tantra and the presence of Tantra communities around the world has introduced sexual healing in informal settings between people who are acquainted but who don't have a personal relationship (i.e. workshop attendees, fellow students, puja ceremony participants, Tantric parties, etc.).

In this book, I am primarily addressing formal sexual healing sessions between trained sexual healers in professional sessions with clients. However, the guidelines and principles for this type of sexual healing also apply to informal and unprofessional sessions with participants who are personally familiar with each other.

Most Importantly

To anyone considering sexual healing: **BEFORE** doing any work with a sexual healer, be clear about the session's *Purpose*, the session's *Container* (activities and their boundary limitations) and establish *Consent* concerning the roles, activities and treatments for the session—and these should be fully considered and clearly understood, and mutually agreed upon. If nothing else, be absolutely clear about these three primary subjects. More elaboration for each subject is presented in later chapters along with suggested ways to achieve clarity on each point.

Sexual Healing or Erotic Enrichment?

The field of sexual healing has many expressions whose treatments range in intimacy and explicitness from PG to R to NC17—to use a movie rating analogy. Concerning the emotional toll or triggering potential, some treatments and activities could be considered mild or "light," with others more involved and emotionally challenging or "heavy." Sexual Healers should consider a client's unique condition and recommend or perform only the treatments that are appropriately suited to their client's needs—including their ability to absorb and integrate their experience.

Throughout this book, I make a distinction between *"sexual healing"* and *"erotic enrichment"* which pertains to differences in the participation and purpose of each type of session. While elements of both can be present in either experience—to promote safe interaction and healthy outcomes aligned with the client's condition and intention it is imperative that the nature of the session be clearly worked out and understood, and mutually agreed upon ahead of time.

Sexual Healing

In general, **sexual healing** pertains to methods of helping survivors of sexual trauma to heal and return to a condition of emotional, physical, and sexual homeostasis, autonomy and empowerment.

Sexual healing sessions fundamentally include *one-way* touch from healer to the client—if any touch between client and healer is present at all in the session. With this type of treatment activity, the healer *gives* and the client *receives*. The sexual healing session is focused on the client and their experience with healing and does not include the healer receiving touch from the client, nor is the healer's personal sexual fulfillment considered or accommodated.

Erotic Enrichment

At least for the purposes of this guidebook, *erotic enrichment* pertains to getting help with experiencing or adding new experience, or stretching into new or uncomfortable areas beyond one's experience with, sexuality and sensuality, and sexual interaction. It can also focus on becoming more empowered and capable with sex, sexual energy, and overcoming blocks to experiencing pleasure and having healthy sexual self-esteem.

For survivors healing sexual trauma, erotic enrichment sessions typically will occur only after significant progress has been made in their healing program. Erotic enrichment sessions are often one-way touch like sexual healing sessions are, but in some cases, and for some practitioners, erotic enrichment sessions can include *mutual touch* activities—with mutual pleasuring that includes the facilitator participating more like a lover would.

Erotic enrichment sessions rarely include intercourse but can often include genital touching during a sensual massage. While an erotic enrichment session may be planned and implemented for a client's benefit, it can also be the case that the session facilitator receives sexual pleasure from their participation in the session.

- **Sexual Healing**: one way touch, healer's pleasure not considered nor is their sexual fulfillment included.
- **Erotic Enrichment**: One way or mutual touch, facilitator's pleasure considered and sexual fulfillment included in some sessions with some facilitators.

The differences between sexual healing and erotic enrichment sessions concern the session activity and participation by the healer and the client; and the potential inclusion of the facilitator's pleasure from mutual touch and pleasure. These differences are significant, and require that additional *carefully considered consent* be reached when an *erotic enrichment type* of session is being planned, and before being implemented in a session. (See section: on Consent)

Caution and additional care should be used when survivors of sexual abuse consider erotic enrichment sessions. The mutual pleasure and mutual touch nature of some erotic enrichment sessions are likely to be too much for a sexual abuse survivor to handle if introduced irresponsibly and prematurely.

Erotic enrichment sessions may be appropriate for some survivors of sexual abuse after they have progressed with their sexual healing program to be able to handle a weightier and more impactful level of sensual activity and feel emotionally ready for the experience.

Why Safer Sexual Healing Practices are Needed Now

There is a growing number of alternative healers, coaches, counselors, therapists, and energy workers who are finding the need to address sexual trauma issues and sexual healing subjects as part of their client's past experience and healing journey. For these healers, therapists, and coaches this guidebook discusses the sexual healer— client dynamic which occurs in sessions and offers guidance on how to handle and support a client's sexual abuse issues effectively and provide support without causing harm.

It also seems that humanity is going through a great catharsis and healing of its collective shadow—and trauma from sexual assault or abuse is at the root of many people's symptoms. For survivors of sexual assault or abuse who are potential clients of sexual healers, this guidebook presents information to help them make informed decisions to get the healing they seek without being harmed in the process. This book is for the many women and men who are survivors of sexual abuse or assault and who want to know:

- What is sexual healing and how does it work?
- What to expect during a sexual healing session.
- How to create boundaries that make you feel safe.
- How to choose a sexual healer.

Tantra

The principles and suggestions in this guidebook also apply to a growing population who have become more comfortable with sexuality and sexual energy through learning about *Tantra*—the ancient esoteric science that includes sex as a path to enlightenment—which is also used as a sexual healing modality today. Tantra is very powerful in uncovering the personal shadow aspects of sexuality and can easily trigger personal issues and wounds around sex—especially sexual abuse. Unless otherwise indicated, whenever Tantra is mentioned I am referring to Western styled neo-Tantra, as distinguished from traditional Tantra as taught by Vajrayana Dzogchen and Kashmir Shaivism lineage schools in the East.

Medical Ethics

Traditional medicine's ethical standards that preclude touching a client's genitals or stimulating their body to activate sexual arousal are there to protect clients from unscrupulous or predatory healers who harm their clients. Yet, many effective sexual healing therapies do include sensual touch and stimulation of these intimate areas of the body for therapeutic healing purposes. (See: Sexual Energy in Therapeutic Healing) Traditional medicine's ethics notwithstanding, the information in this guidebook is intended to enhance and encourage protection of a client's safety and wellbeing and to positively inform the sexual healer-client relationship.

This guidebook is for informational purposes only—with the intention of sponsoring responsible consideration and conscientious implementation of safer sexual healing practices. No part of this guidebook is intended to replace or preclude regular medical treatment and practice by a qualified physician or therapist. This guidebook aspires to the highest ethical standards while preserving a client's right to choose what therapies and treatments are appropriate for them; and that clients are responsibly informed regarding treatment methods and therapies that are included in a sexual healing session.

LGBTQ+

Sexual abuse and emotional trauma are experienced by people of any and all genders and sexual identification. The principles of safety and best practices that promote positive transformation, healing, and a return to a sense of wellbeing equally apply to any gender or sex identification. Ultimately what matters most is the healer's care and consideration of their client's personal experience and what their unique needs are for healing. Try to find a sexual healer who you feel most comfortable with and who understands your gender and sexual identification to your satisfaction.

I have had several gay and a few transgender clients and feel great compassion for marginalized communities who are underrepresented in social dialogue and in sexual healing topics. In writing this book I have tried to use inclusive pronouns, however, I realize that some descriptions are hetero-normative and cisgendered in viewpoint. I apologize for any offense anyone may feel or any sense of diminishment that this may create for some readers.

Sexual Healing and Wellbeing

Wellness is subjectively felt and includes many areas of life and experiences with people and circumstances. However, in general, a sense of wellbeing comes from physical, mental, spiritual, emotional and social wellness or homeostasis—everything feels OK, or better.

For many people, wellbeing also includes the state of their experience of sexuality and their sensual, body-mind-emotion integration. Sexual trauma has a severe impact on sexual experience and the body-mind-emotion connection. So addressing symptoms that impact or limit an unencumbered experience of sexuality or a fluent sensual body-mind-emotion connection falls under sexual healing in pursuit of wellbeing.

Trauma and Wellbeing

The healthy human set point is a state of mental flexibility, emotional openness, dynamically creative, and responsive to inspiration or purpose. Trauma survivors can often feel: reactive, insecure, fearful, contracted, stuck, disconnected, closed, blocked, disempowered, and depressed.

The effects of trauma cause a complex enmeshment and knotting of mental-emotional energy. Trauma creates an emotional overwhelm and produces beliefs or judgments which have negative emotional, mental, and physical effects that numb sensation and limit pleasure.

Unresolved sexual trauma is a major influence in a survivor's life—even if they aren't consciously aware of it. Trauma takes a toll on a person's energy and creative spark. It can dim the hope of their life getting better and can make depression and self-abusive behavior more likely.

Most Important—Do No Harm

No more important a tenant of sexual healing could there be than to *not cause harm to those whom you are helping heal.* The concept of **harmlessness** was articulated as long ago as the 8th century B.C.E. in Vedic texts as the spiritual principle of "*Ahimsa*." Ahimsa is a Sanskrit term that means to "do no harm" (literally: the avoidance of violence – *himsa*) and is an important tenet of the Indian religions: Hinduism, Buddhism and especially Jainism.[1]

Sexual Healers work with a client's most sensitive and intimate core concerns and challenges to their self-esteem or worthiness, and their emotional and physical vulnerability. It is therefore essential that a sexual healer understands and implements the principle of *ahimsa*.

The emotional, physical and psychological intimacy associated with the sexual healing process requires impeccable integrity with maintaining harmlessness. A sexual healer must steward each session with the utmost respect, care, and concern for the client's wellbeing and safety while supporting their unique pace and ability to absorb and integrate their experience.

Sexual Healing

The need for sexual healing comes from the pervasive sexual abuse and assault that is prevalent throughout modern culture. It's a huge problem that modern medicine has few answers for—with most medical practices and disciplines inadequately able to address the subject of survivors' sexual trauma symptoms.

Sexual abuse and assault are widely believed to be underreported crimes because of the stigma involved and the self-doubt of victims who may wrongly blame themselves. One recent public health study released by the Centers for Disease Control and Prevention estimated that 23 million women in the U.S. have been raped during their lifetime. Another survey run by the Bureau of Justice Statistics estimated that there were about 174,000 victims of rapes and sexual assaults in 2012. Child sexual abuse is also suspected of being underreported, with some studies estimating that 1 in 20 children have been abused in the UK and as many as 1 in 5 girls and 1 in 20 boys the victims of child sexual abuse in the US.

What is Sexual Healing?

Sexual healing is the facilitation of healing from sexual and emotional trauma effecting a person's sexuality and their ability to experience sexual intimacy fluently. It is also a methodology that uses sexual energy as a therapeutic tool to evaluate and treat symptoms. And, it is a healing practice that frequently involves the sexual body and its pleasure centers.

Sexual healing has existed for centuries in traditional and alternative healing modalities that treat the types of symptoms that survivors of sexual abuse deal with. However, these modalities and their treatments might not have been thought of as "sexual healing" per se. Yet, they address similar symptoms that sexual healing does: physiological conditions like genital pain, stiffness, and diminished sensitivity, emotional and psychological conditions that impact sexuality, arousal and sexual performance, libido, or impotence; as well as relationship issues dealing with sexual compatibility and communication, and overcoming sexual issues within a relationship.

What is new in recent decades is a formalized profession of *sexual healers* and the inclusion of sensual somatic activation— physically touching the client to stimulate and utilize sexual energy therapeutically. Sexual healing is both a unique and powerful opportunity; having an incredible potential for genuine healing as well as significant exposure to harm if not practiced conscientiously and with ethical integrity.

Physical healing involves many things like repairing tissue, setting bones, removing viruses, and promoting the optimal functioning of organs, muscles, glands, etc. Sexual healing, however, involves restoration or development of sensual integration and sexual embodiment—the ability to fully experience and express oneself sexually without encumbrance or blocks. Sexual healing specifically addresses the mental-emotional-somatic-energetic symptoms felt by survivors of sexual abuse/assault.

Sexual healing can also address sexual empowerment and the integration and transparency of emotions felt with sexual expression and experience. Healthy sexuality has an organic and synergistic mind-body-heart connection—with sexual energy flowing organically and naturally. Sexual healing sessions can help a client repair, restore or improve this connection and establish ease and fluency in their sexual experience.

As a modality addressing a client's issues and symptoms, *"sexual healing* is different than *sex counseling*. Where *sexual healing* treatments and sessions can include some amount of disrobing by the client, explicit demonstrations, and/or touching the client by the practitioner; *sex counseling* does not include any of these." [2]

Sexual healing works at the *psychoid* [3] (psycho-somatic) level of experience—bridging the psychological and physical. This means that sexual healing methods normally have both an emotional-psychological component combined with physical and sensual elements. The sexual healing process usually includes some amount of discovery, acceptance, processing, integrating, and releasing of trauma emotions and addressing the client's associated energetic and somatic symptoms. Sexual healing reconnects and reestablishes the optimal function and natural flow of the client's sexual energy. This is accomplished by helping a client recognize and remove—or unwind their emotional and energetic "knots" that prevent them from experiencing an integrated and fluent sexual expression and experience.

Benefits of Sexual Healing

Sexual healing sessions provide a safe container to discover, release, grow, heal, explore and become sensually/sexually empowered. They are a place to safely process and learn more about the feelings, beliefs, and limitations associated with the symptoms of sexual trauma. The result of healing sexual trauma is a return to a sense of wholeness and well-being. Sexual healing facilitates a client's reconnection to their sexual energy and restores a positive outlook on life.

The benefits of sexual healing include:

Physical: an increased and enhanced sensual-somatic awareness and sensory sensitivity and capacity—promoting a healthy mind-body-emotion integration.

Emotional: an expanded sense of wellbeing and cohesive emotional integration; and enhanced awareness of emotional presence and connection with present experience.

Mental: an enhanced cognitive awareness and processing ability; including the ability to remain present with present sensual, physical, and emotional experience without dissociation, overwhelm or fragmentation.

Spiritual: an expanded consciousness and enhanced awareness of spiritual connection, and more sensitivity to subtle energy and numinous experience.

Sexual: a fluent experience and expression of sexual energy and desire, creating more sexual fulfillment.

Addressing Symptoms

Disorders associated with sexual trauma stemming from sexual abuse, molestation or assault have psychological, emotional, physical and energetic symptoms that affect sexual desire, arousal, interaction, and orgasm, as well as the ability to feel and sustain emotional intimacy and connection. A survivor desires to heal their body-mind-emotion integration and be able to feel and enjoy sex without discomfort, pain, numbness, self-judgment, fear, or dissociation. Also, a survivor's symptoms are capable of effecting additional areas of life in the form of low energy, low self-esteem, blocked creativity, depression, and a negative outlook. Healing and restoring the flow of sexual energy to a more organic and natural expression restores a brighter personal outlook with more vitality and energy, happiness and general sense of wellbeing.

The physical body is a repository for emotional wounds which are *imprinted* in memory and embedded in the body locus—usually in areas which are near, at, or refer to places where the sexual abuse occurred. Sexual healing treatments address the physical aspect of knotted sexual energy in the body by purposely including sensual and somatic treatments in the healing process. Treatments that relax the body, like conscious breathing, massage and acupressure, body movement, and sensual touch activation, assist in discovering the psycho-somatic locations of trauma and in releasing their restricted or blocked energy.

The degree of sensual touch and physical intimacy experienced in a sexual healing session may vary from *off-the-body* no-touch to *hands-on* treatments that include sensual massage—or sometimes invasive procedures such as internal pelvic release (manual vaginal/anal penetration). Knowing the degree of sexual touch to be experienced in a session is a vital part of informed consent that should be discussed prior to engaging in the session (See section: on **Consent**).

Sexual healing takes time and usually is not a *quick fix* remedy. Multiple sessions are often necessary to establish an effective level of trust that's needed between sexual healer and client to work through layers of armoring before genuine and lasting healing can take place. Promises of miraculous, quick fixes should be suspect and caution should be taken to avoid being harmed by a reckless or unscrupulous healer.

The Body-Mind Nexus

A modern pioneer of sexual healing was Dr. Wilhelm Reich (1897 – 1957). An Austrian psychoanalyst, he argued that neurosis is rooted in physical, sexual and socio-economic conditions, and in particular in a lack of what he called "orgastic potency" [sic]. Reich believed that the repression of original trauma was maintained by the suppression of sexual feeling. This suppression predisposed the client to symptoms that were triggered by subsequent sexual engagement. To Reich, the client's psychological neurosis was the root cause of overt symptoms that included a physical-sexual correspondence; and a person's attitude and relationship to sexuality predisposed an individual to neurotic symptoms. He proposed that muscular armoring, or chronic muscular tensions, serve to maintain the client's condition by binding sexual energy so that it cannot be discharged—limiting sexual excitement. To Reich, a healthy individual would have no such limitation, and their energy would not be bound in muscular armoring. A healthy individual's energy would be readily available for sexual pleasure or any other creative expression.[4]

One of Reich's students, Alexander Lowen, M.D., (1910 – 2008) took his theories further and created a new treatment modality called *Bioenergetics* that combined physical touch with psychological observation. [5] Lowen explains the connection between touch and helping clients to heal by asserting that the avoidance of touching in traditional psychoanalysis places *"a barrier between two people who needed to be in touch with each other more immediately than through words. By touching a patient's body, a therapist can sense many things about him. Through his touch, he can convey to the patient the idea that he feels and accepts the patient as a bodily being and that touching is a natural way of being in contact."*

Lowen suggests that when a client is touched physically by the therapist, it shows that the therapist cares and harkens back to the days when being held and touched by one's mother was an expression of her tender, loving care. He asserts that touch deprivation is rampant in modern society and that it is therapeutically important to eliminate this taboo—writing: *"It is incumbent on a therapist, therefore, to show he is not afraid to touch or be in touch with his patient."* [6]

In sexual healing, the touch between practitioner and client may go beyond what Reich or Lowen advocated. In fact, Dr. Lowen emphatically warns against the sexual touch of a therapist to a patient, writing that it would reinforce the patient's deep anxiety about physical touch. However, I suggest that Lowen's objection is about personal sexual interaction and doesn't consider the professional, therapeutic application of sexual energy that is present in today's sexual healing. For many clients who feel ready for sexual healing and who work with conscientious and considerate healers in a container of informed consent, there is a great opportunity to accomplish the healing they seek.

Any client should only receive treatments appropriate to their ability to integrate their experience. Abundant caution should be taken to ensure appropriate treatment when a client has a high degree of emotional and psychological fragility or woundedness. These clients are likely best served by talk-only therapy until/if they become ready for hands-on treatments. If someone has doubts about working with a hands-on sexual healer, it's a good indication that they are not ready to do so yet and should work with a traditional "talk" therapist or a *sans-touch* healer until they feel ready to go further—and only *if* they feel it is desirable for them to do so.

Sexual Healing's Contemporary Development

In recent years, schools for clinical sexology and sexological bodywork have been established to provide a contemporary platform for responsible sexual healing training and the ethical application of sexual healing treatments. (See Appendix for list)

A recent contribution to the field of body-based psychotherapy is the work of therapist Peter A. Levine—which he calls "Somatic Experiencing." [7] His methods seek to treat post-traumatic stress and other mental and physical trauma-related health issues by promoting awareness and release of physical tension associated with trauma. Somatic Experiencing includes some engagement with the body, however, as a stand-alone treatment it does not include genital stimulation. Sexual Healers might use somatic experiencing as complementary to other treatments in sexual healing sessions.

With the advances in the understanding of the body-mind connection and the role of the unconscious in healing and wellbeing, competent *hands-on* sexual healing treatment is now available from trained and certified practitioners. I think that both Reich and Lowen would approve of the appropriately trained, qualified and responsible application of the current treatments typically used in sexual healing in a container that is well-considered and consented to.

Sexual Healing, not Personal Sex

Personal sexual engagement is not the same as the therapeutic application of sexual energy. (See the section: Sexual Energy in Therapeutic Healing) As long as the healing practitioner maintains a therapeutic container and engagement, sexual healing can be effective and beneficial for the client. In the same way that a massage therapist can touch a client's body and maintain therapeutic intent and emotional containment to provide a therapeutic service—so can a qualified and conscientious sexual healer serve their client.

The form that sexual healing sessions take can vary widely. Some healers might not touch their client's body at all—with both the client and healer remaining fully clothed. Most sexual healers will remain clothed and the client only partially exposed depending on the treatment being used. Other healers might be fully or partially undressed (See section: **Nudity in a Session**), and at one end of the spectrum under some circumstances some sexual healers might engage in sexual contact with a client—which can include intercourse.

That being said, my impression of what is commonly practiced by most sexual healers is they:

- Don't have sex with clients
- With consent, will touch a client's body applying *hands-on healing* treatments
- Will provide treatments while being fully clothed

It's extremely important that both client and sexual healer discuss ahead of time how the healing session will be structured and what treatments will be included.

How Does Sexual Healing Work?

Sexual abuse trauma creates a *knot* or contraction in sexual energy which is felt both physically and emotionally. This clenched knot has the ability to suppress feeling experience and restrict the flow of life force energy—especially in sensual experience.

When a sexual abuse survivor is exposed to situations that trigger their trauma wounds—a maladaptive stress reaction occurs affecting their mood and disposition; including possible emotional overwhelm. According to Dr. Darren Weissman, a maladaptive stress reaction occurs *"when one is not able to adapt in the present moment, our body reacts as if something from the past is going on right now."* For a sexual abuse survivor in that state, it is as if they are on some level reliving the trauma of their experience—which causes great distress and disruption.

Sexual healing addresses a client's trauma symptoms and condition by unwinding or detangling the energetic and emotional knots created by sexual trauma. The sexual healing process reveals where a client's sexual energy knots exist on a psycho-somatic level; and then treats their condition and the symptoms that the knots have created. Its methods encourage releasing of the physical and emotional armoring of the knotted sexual energy to restore optimum availability and flow to fluent sexual expression and experience.

Therapeutically Applied Pleasure

Sensual pleasure unleashes elevated levels of oxytocin (the "cuddle hormone" [8]) which makes the subject feel dreamy waves of bliss. Research shows that oxytocin increases emotional connection and promotes a state of calm wellbeing, reducing the effects of stress and pain. Additional neurochemicals released during sensual pleasure are endorphins which are a natural painkiller; generating elation and euphoria. [9]

Sexual abuse trauma will create contractions or obstructions of pleasure signals and these are felt by a client as actual physical locations in, or on the body—often where past trauma has occurred. These places can feel numb or can be *trigger points*, knots of energy, which can have strong emotions, judgments or memories attached to them. These places can also refer to other locations on the body where similar symptoms are present. Therapeutically applied pleasure helps to release the sexual energy knots and their strong emotions and restore physical sensation and emotional integration.

Sexual healing sessions often employ sensual pleasure to encourage and sustain erotic excitation. Accessing a combined state of relaxation and erotic excitation provides relief from stress and tension and promotes homeostasis—*"everything is OK"*—improving wellbeing. This relief is important for sexual abuse survivors who can be stuck in a state of chronic anxiety. Pleasure can improve outlook, self-esteem and sexual empowerment, and works to create a positive and healthy body-mind-emotion integration.

In addition, by creating a unique combination of deep relaxation and erotic excitation a client's psycho-somatic armoring and emotional barriers are softened to allow deeper layers of trauma to be accessed and released. This state also allows for sensual rehabilitation, reconditioning, and a reestablishing of sensorial pathways that *pleasure map* the body.

Sexual Energy in Therapeutic Healing

Most adults are used to experiencing sexual energy within a committed relationship, in a private setting, and only with their partner. So, it may seem strange to consider that sexual energy can be used therapeutically to facilitate healing.

When properly considered, prepared, and facilitated, the client's activated sexual energy creates a state of mind and body that feels at ease, excited, and enlivened. A *therapeutic* application means that the sexual energy, erotic excitement, and pleasure are being created to facilitate the client's healing—not to promote a personal sexual relationship between healer and client. Clients feel safe when they are confident that the healer – client relationship boundaries won't be crossed and they can focus on their experience and their process of healing without personal complications.

Once activated, erotic, sexual energy begins reconnecting and restoring vibrancy and wellbeing. Sexual energy enlivens and excites the body as it creates new experiences of aliveness and sexual fluency.

Activated sexual energy will also bring up a client's emotional and psychological "shadow issues" from sexual abuse trauma. Sensual pleasure associated with activated sexual energy can bring relief from symptoms or conditions but this is usually only temporary relief if deeper trauma healing work is not also included in the client's healing program. Not everyone needs deep shadow work to feel relief, and for those that need shadow work—not all are ready for it. Care with applying pleasure at an appropriate level for an individual client is essential.

Sexual healing is not for everybody and receiving pleasure and activating sexual energy is not always appropriate for some sexual abuse survivors with sexual trauma. (See section: The Client) For some survivors of sexual abuse, receiving pleasure is not only difficult or confusing, the experience can overwhelm them and trigger a stress reaction and emotional shock which is counterproductive and can cause harm.

Care and caution should always be taken by anyone considering sexual healing to make sure they feel ready to pursue it and they are resolved that it is something they want to experience to facilitate their healing. As mentioned earlier, survivors having difficulties with severe trauma symptoms should consult with a therapist before seeking sexual healing.

Activating Sexual Energy without Sexual Intercourse

In sexual healing sessions, activating sexual energy does not mean that sexual intercourse or other sexual activities are necessary. Sexual energy can be activated by using *breathing or movement exercises* that don't include erotic touch.

Potential clients should ask healers in pre-session consultations if sensual touch will be included in the session and if so, where and how it will be applied, and for what purpose. Responsibly using sexual energy in therapeutic healing means that the healer considers the uniqueness of their client's condition and tailors session treatments appropriately.

Activated sexual energy, therapeutically applied, is used both as an evaluation tool and as a type of healing treatment. Some of the ways sexual energy is considered during healing sessions are:

- As an observable ability to feel and experience sexual energy—to access, have awareness of, and be responsive to sexual energy and see how fluently integrated it is with somatic sensation and emotional clarity.

- As an aspect of treatments that shows where on the body there is a block, contraction, or restriction that diminishes or turns off sensation or connection to sexual energy and to what or where it refers to—other physical locations, thoughts, emotions, or memories.

- As a metaphysical *healing elixir* with the power to transform and reconnect disparate psychic, emotional and sensual aspects and restore energy flow. This may seem *"out there"* to some, however, there is no doubt that activated sexual energy experienced as *pleasure* can be healing for many symptoms and conditions.

Impacted sexual energy manifests as interruptions in the mind-body-emotion integration and indicates the presence of the effects of emotional trauma. The client's inability to feel somatic sensation, emotion, or to stay present with pleasure experience can manifest as symptoms of low libido, emotional fragmentation, physical numbness, psychological dissociation, and intervening thoughts, memories, or images.

One method used in sexual healing is to observe a client's sexual arousal cycle and notice when and where there are *"glitches,"* or breaks in the flow of their experience. Wherever an interruption occurs is an opportunity to discover what contributing thoughts, beliefs, or unconscious patterns are being triggered—and reveal their root causes.

Sexual energy itself has a profound power to heal and transform. If appropriately facilitated by a trained and competent sexual healer, it can work to reconnect and improve debilitated conditions. Clients who might otherwise not be able to feel or activate their sexual energy can, with the aid of a sexual healer, transcend limitations they are not able to by themselves.

Sexual Healing, is it Legal?

Due to the intimate nature of sexual healing sessions, uninformed or skeptical communities have trepidation and great concern for the protection and welfare of their citizens. The great fear they have is that clients of sexual healing will be exposed to unscrupulous or reckless healers who will cause harm to them. Unfortunately, there have been some "bad apples" who justify these concerns and have brought dishonor to the sexual healing profession.

Depending on where you are in the world, sexual healing may be completely acceptable and legal—or considered to be illegal sex work, like prostitution. Even in areas where it is not legal, there can be tacit acceptance as long as it occurs between consenting adults and there is no accusation of harm resulting from the experience.

My personal opinion is that most authorities have better things to spend their department's budget on and time policing, and unless a complaint is made, law enforcement officials won't go after sexual healers who don't flout community standards or salaciously market themselves as providing sex services. I believe that in the areas where sexual healing is not expressly legal, if the practitioner maintains a respectable public profile and responsibly promotes their service as *education* or *alternative healing*—and not as a thinly veiled form of prostitution—they will most likely be left alone unless complaints are made.

Sexual Healers are located all across the US and in many countries around the world. Depending on where you live, it may be easy or very difficult to find a sexual healer to work with due to their need to work *"under the radar"* to avoid being persecuted or prosecuted. My hope is that in harmony with what this book promotes there will be a movement towards greater openness and acceptance in more areas of the world where sexual healing can thrive and bring its positive effects to more communities.

For sexual trauma survivors and their healers who are sincerely seeking the client's healing by working together within consented boundaries and activities, there should be no reason to be in fear of law enforcement—if care is taken and no harm occurs.

Fundamentals for Sexual Healing

The Healing Alliance

The healing alliance describes the *right-relationship* between the sexual healing facilitator and the client that produces and maintains a therapeutic container where transformative healing can safely and harmlessly take place. The healing alliance is an understanding between the client and the healer concerning the roles and responsibilities each possesses and contributes during a healing session.

The sexual healer contributes to the healing alliance by *maintaining a therapeutic container that supports the client's intention of transformation and healing* and which respects the client's boundaries. The therapeutic container for a healing session or program of treatment includes the physical, energetic, and emotional boundaries for interaction and activities agreed upon by the client and healer. The healer's role in the healing alliance is to gently steward their client's process of healing, and reconnecting to or remembering wholeness and wellbeing.

The client participates in the healing alliance by meeting the healer in the space of possibility (to release/let go, transform and heal) with *informed participation* seeking to return to wholeness and wellbeing. During a session, the client contributes by reporting their state of being and their needs/desires, which helps the sexual healer know where the client is at emotionally and to keep the session current with the client's consent. Each must trust the other to fulfill their respective roles as conscientiously as possible.

Fundamental to the healing alliance is clear and informed **consent**. Without consent, sexual healing session activities are likely to have adverse consequences and can potentially harm the client.

Consent

Consent is an essential concept to be clear on in order for safe sexual healing to take place. The Merriam-Webster dictionary defines consent as "to agree to do or allow something: to give permission for something to happen or be done." And, "to be in concord in opinion or sentiment." [10]

Clearly, the intent of *consent* is to determine mutual understanding and agreement about an interaction or experience; where both parties are *on the same page*. Going further than merely permitting something to happen, consent seeks to establish the intent or purpose for an activity so a more clear understanding and agreement are possible. This kind of consent includes who is doing what to whom and how it will be implemented in the session within the bounds of the consented activity.

Consent in a sexual healing context requires careful consideration of the client's authentic feelings—their truth about their current state, their desire for, and their ability to handle treatments. With sexual healing, consent needs to be more than simply *allowing something to happen*—it must go further to provide a *clear understanding* of session activities and boundaries and come to a considered and settled decision to participate.

Consent is about respecting, honoring, valuing, and empowering the client. It directly bears on the healing session's container of activities and boundaries and includes agreeing on what activities will happen in a session and which ones will not. Consent also addresses the expectations and intention of a session as well as establishing what to do when there is a need to stop or slow down or change an activity. The sexual healer will lead the healing session but the client's input and ongoing consent are vitally important to guiding the session and preventing harm from occurring.

Sometimes if consent is not adequately considered or not given enough importance, clients can bypass their feelings and attempt to tolerate an activity they don't really feel in consent with. Sexual abuse survivors can have an impaired ability to access their true feelings and can feel overwhelmed by their emotional wounds. This is why it is so important for consent to be reached after a careful consideration that satisfies the client's concerns and questions, and which results in their settled resolve.

During a session, consent must remain current with the client's ability to handle or process their experience, and accommodate any change in desire they may have at the moment. If there is a change in a client's consent, the client should make it known immediately and a new container with different or new activities and boundaries worked out. If this occurs, the healer should allow for as much time as the client needs to adjust and reestablish consent.

Consent helps a sexual healer know what their client is feeling during a session and avoids making assumptions that could unintentionally cause harm. When consent is considered and enacted consciously it evokes the client's feelings of personal respect, consideration, and empowerment which will help rehabilitate their sense of autonomy, personal value, and worthiness.

Creating a Container of Consent

Creating the container for sexual healing includes considering and determining the limitations and boundaries of activities and treatments to be included in a healing session, and is something that must be done together—with input from both client and healer. Arrangements should be made for a consent discussion before starting any sessions (and preferably not right before a session) to allow a client enough time for considering their concerns and to process the information provided by the sexual healer.

Clearly understood boundaries gives a client the assurance of autonomy (a key aspect of selfhood that is often damaged by sexual abuse) and enables them to participate as an equal partner in the healing process—wholeheartedly engaging instead of submitting to something that is *done to them.*

A lack of clear boundaries creates confusion and can invite opportunities for emotional harm—with the client feeling like they have been assaulted. Clients want to heal and let go of what's limiting their sexual experience and emotional connection, and recover from trauma to feel whole again—not add to their wounds with more trauma created in a sexual healing session.

Sexual Healers also need to provide their consent and need to be clear on their boundaries and disclose these to their client. In determining their boundaries, they must be able to contain any personal issues or triggers that would otherwise divert a session from being about the client's healing process to being about the healer's personal issues. To deviate from an agreed upon consent container and pursue personal gratification agendas crosses boundaries and contaminates the container of the healing session.

Get Clear on All Activities to be Included in a Session

The sexual healer should initiate a discussion to discover what a client desires to work on and inform them of the possible treatments and activities –and their likely effects– which address their symptoms and intention to heal. The purpose of this discussion is to provide ample information that the client will consider and then share their feelings about and comfort level with.

Answers to questions like "What is this activity intended to do?" and "How will this treatment help me with my symptoms?" will provide valuable information for a client to consider. This discussion should also include details like whether or not session activities and treatments include touching a client and if so, where and for what purpose?

In the consent discussion about session activities and treatments, the healer must use discernment and listen for where the client's *edge* is—what would be *too much* for the client to handle in their present condition. This information establishes an unexpressed boundary where the healer is conscious of their client's sensitivity and ability to safely process and contain their experience. Stretching or going beyond this edge should only happen with extreme care and never impromptu or haphazardly.

Sexual Healers should be able to monitor and discern a client's disposition and keep the session on track without it going beyond what the client can handle. Sessions should include many opportunities for checking-in with a client as well as monitoring their experience and encouraging them to speak up any time they feel something is too much or *is out of consent* for them.

Here are some things to include and consider when establishing consent boundaries for healing sessions:

- Discuss the client's desire and intention for healing, and what subjects and areas of concern or challenge will be addressed during sessions.
- Understand a client's symptoms and how these are impacting their experience.

- Discuss the activities for a session including who will be doing what to whom? And, what type of touch will be used, and where?
- Understand the intent and purpose of agreed upon activities for a session.
- Encourage free and open disclosure and owning of feelings without consequences of shame, judgment, or guilt.
- Support frank and honest discussion of the client's vulnerability and where their edge of feeling safe and in consent is anytime during the session.
- Ask for and receive feedback frequently, in discussion before or during a session that effectively maintains wholehearted consent participation.

Major shifts in the session's container, boundaries, activity progression, or the introduction of new activities or treatments that stretch the client's edge of feeling safe should be given sufficient discussion before being included *in a future session* to allow for the client's full consideration and wholehearted participation.

Working with a Client's Edge

In many cases, healing or growth requires a client to stretch past their current comfort level which is keeping them from where they want to be. A client's edge also includes their level of tolerance for pleasure or their ability to receive it readily—desiring to, while yet experiencing encumbrances or blocks to doing so. Their edge also concerns their ability to assimilate their experience and integrate session treatments.

With sexual healing, working with a client's edge is especially sensitive and care is needed to prevent harm from occurring. Once boundaries are set, and the activities and treatments to be used during a session are agreed upon, *further discussion about gently stretching the client's edge* should also take place. This conversation would include aspects of session treatments like length of time, progression of application, expanding or widening areas or scope of treatments, and other ways in which the client's edge might be engaged and worked with. The healer will want to rely heavily on the client's input and feedback on this subject—and especially during session treatments—to gauge the activity/treatment facilitation, alteration, or its completion.

Session activities should be designed to support a client's healing or growth which can be challenging and take them near their edge. Discuss and establish how -in relation to the activities and boundaries agreed upon- the client's experience might be *stretched* and make clear that either the healer or client should intervene if it is felt the stretch is too much for the client to handle.

Consent and Sexual Healing treatments

In sexual healing, consent begins with a thorough understanding of the client's current emotional condition, previous sexual abuse experiences, and current trauma symptoms. It is important to know where the client has the potential for emotional sensitivity, reactiveness, or *acute stress reaction* triggers and be prepared for these potentials.

Sexual healing sessions usually follow a typical practitioner-client model where session activities and treatments are applied in a one-way direction with the client receiving treatment from the sexual healer. To effectively accomplish this, a sexual abuse survivor must have complete trust that their healer will abide by the consent worked out earlier and will maintain professional and ethical integrity throughout the session.

Sexual abuse survivors need to know that their boundaries will be respected before they feel safe enough to open up to sexual healing treatments. Their reactive and often hyper-sensitive feelings can be quickly triggered and overwhelmed and cause emotional harm. If a sexual healing session were to have undisclosed treatments or unexpectedly include mutual pleasuring or bi-directional touch it could easily confuse and overwhelm a survivor of sexual trauma.

Consent necessitates that all pertinent information bearing on session activities be disclosed and considered, and that consent be the backbone of all interactions and conversations with clients. Consent needs to be pervasive and never be assumed—even for apparently *light* sessions that aren't intended to have a heavy emotional impact.

If in doubt, ask. If a sexual healer has any question or doubts about a client's emotional state or with their readiness to experience a treatment, they should pause and check-in with the client. Also, there should be an expectation and standing invitation during a session for the client to assertively interject and disclose any change in consent that they feel.

Maintaining Consent during a Session

Some healers might feel it can be a hindrance and distraction to implement consent during a session. However, once rapport and trust have been established an easy and flowing way of checking-in without disrupting the flow of the session is possible. A sexual healer whose mind is *present and aware* should notice multiple places where checking-in is appropriate. This will reassure the client that they are in control and provide the basis for their consent to be ongoing and current.

During the healing session, the sexual healer watches for signs of disturbance in their client (dissociating, tensing, clenching, holding breath) and notes what is happening and takes the opportunity to ask the client what thoughts or feelings have come up. After addressing these the sexual healer can gently re-establish the intent and direction of the session and ask for the client's feelings about continuing the activity—waiting for their response to proceed.

Examples of checking consent during a session could include asking "How are you feeling?" or "What came up for you just now?" After allowing some time for the client to gather their thoughts and feelings, and listening to their response, the sexual healer provides feedback or support and then checks-in about consent. "How do you feel about continuing with this activity?"

During a session, there will also be organic breaks after and between treatments or exercises where checking in about the client's emotional state and consent are appropriate. At these opportunities, healers can ask questions similar to the above.

Without ensuring that consent is maintained during a session the gulf between the client's *experience* and the provider's intention can be immense and invites possible harm rather than facilitating an effective and transformational healing experience.

Clarifying the Intention and Purpose of a Session

An essential part of establishing consent is knowing what the intention or purpose of a session is and what will be addressed by the activities in the session. Based on the chosen container for a session, there can be various types and levels of activity that will impact and effect clients differently.

If the intention is to address the symptoms of surviving sexual or emotional trauma which is having an impact on sexual experience or relating sexually between partners—then sexual healing sessions are appropriate. These sessions have their own characteristics, activities, and type of participation that make healing sessions safer for survivors.

If the intention is to expand one's comfort zone, to grow in experience or learn and become adept with sensual ability or sexual energy—and if sexual abuse issues or wounds have been addressed and worked with already—then erotic enrichment sessions could be appropriate. These sessions have different consent considerations for activities, boundaries, and kinds of interactions.

Without addressing and making progress with a client's sexual trauma issues first, it's not a good idea to mix the two types of sessions. Mixing sexual healing with erotic enrichment can unintendedly cause harm to sexual trauma survivors. After making enough progress with their healing, erotic enrichment is a valuable and necessary step for survivors to take on their path to wholeness and sexual empowerment when they are ready for it.

Erotic Enrichment

Not all sessions are about sexual healing nor do they involve deeply reactive emotional wounds from sexual abuse. Some are about providing rehabilitation and rejuvenation through experiencing, exploring, practicing, or discovering types of activities. A client might seek to have a sensually enriching experience without a lot of emotional challenge, stretching, or transformation—one that helps them overcome a limitation or to understand something better or to discover something new. This type of session is known as an *erotic enrichment* session, which is normally distinctly different in focus and intention.

The main difference between sexual healing and erotic enrichment sessions is that some erotic enrichment practitioners include mutual pleasuring or touch during session activities with clients. Consent becomes even more vital and complex when mutual pleasuring or bi-directional touch is included between the client and facilitator.

Due to the potential for harm, mutual pleasuring or bi-directional touch is not appropriate for many if not most sexual trauma survivors until significant sexual healing has been reached. However, after significant progress, integration, and healing—*and when a client feels completely ready*—erotic enrichment sessions can be appropriate and very beneficial for reclaiming wholeness and empowerment.

Types of Erotic Enrichment Sessions

Erotic Enrichment sessions seek to replace previous limitations with new abilities and revitalizing experiences. Erotic enrichment sessions can help clients feel more confident in and competent with their sexual energy.

It's important to know that not all erotic enrichment sessions include mutual touch, nor is it necessary that they do. Erotic enrichment sessions exercise sexual energy and often focus on sensual embodiment for maximum integration and fluency of the client's body-mind-emotion connection.

One common form of erotic enrichment session is known as a *full body sensual massage* (FBSM) which often includes a "happy ending"—orgasm. In these sessions, the client receives a full body massage that usually includes stimulation of the pleasure areas of the body. Sensual massage sessions are often focused on improving the client's ability to sensually *receive and feel* while allowing their sexual energy to run undistracted by reciprocal pleasuring.

Here are some examples of women's needs and concerns that can be addressed in erotic enrichment sessions: (paraphrased from actual clients)

- A single woman without a partner has had health problems and hasn't been in a relationship for a long time. She has gained a lot of weight and has worked hard to bring her body back to what feels better, losing weight and feeling more alive again. She is interested in erotic enrichment sessions to reconnect with her body and her sexual energy before seeking an intimate partner to have sex with. She is also interested in learning Tantric practices so when she begins a new relationship she can bring unique new skills to their lovemaking. Her interests are in experiencing and reconnecting with her sexual energy and her body from a new perspective in the safety of sessions with a facilitator who can remain objective and professional.

- A woman is going through major life shifts in her relationship, workplace, and living situation and seeks to come back to herself by discovering her Eros at a deeper, more illuminated level. Her emotions and sexual energy has been shut down for many hears and she wants to heal her issues in a safe context with a man who can be present and show up for her and help her discover more of who she is while facilitating her healing and releasing of the issues which have shut her down.

- A woman's husband has died a few years ago. She has grieved his loss and is now ready for a relationship again. She wants to prepare herself to be with a man's energy and be open to his touch in a safe setting. She also knows that there is likely more to heal and grieve as she opens up to her sexual energy once again and wants to do that with someone who knows how to hold the space and support her through it.

"Daka" and Tantric Date Sessions

Another form of erotic enrichment session is known as a "Daka/Dakini session," or *Tantric date*. Many Tantra practitioners are aware that Tantric sexual energy practices can be healing and help others have a fuller sexual experience by removing energetic and emotional blocks. It's also possible that symptoms which impact sexual energy and experience can be triggered during Tantric practices and during activities which activate sexual energy. The triggering of these symptoms can cause acute stress reaction and be upsetting or cause emotional harm to participants.

In erotic enrichment sessions in the Tantra community, a "Daka" (male Tantric adept) or "Dakini" (female Tantric adept) will engage with a client or student to teach or demonstrate Tantric practices to help them have a Tantric experience. In these sessions, various Tantric energy techniques can be utilized and in some specific cases, these can include mutual touch and pleasuring.

A slightly different version of this is a session between two Tantrikas (Tantra practitioners) sometimes called a "Tantric Date" which is for a similar purpose of gaining experience and practice with using Tantra energy techniques, as well as for healing or for letting go of blockages to sexual energy flow. Like other erotic enrichment sessions, these can have one-direction or mutual touch activities as part of the session.

These Daka/Dakini or Tantric Date sessions might also be focused on sexual healing treatments, and in so doing there can be vagary, recklessness or confusion about boundaries for session activities and the session's purpose. When assumptions are made and no clear communication or consent is discussed it exposes participants to being harmed. Make sure that anytime activities involve activated sexual energy or sexual healing methods that all participants are clear on the session's boundaries and purpose; monitor compliance with those boundaries and speak up if activities are going in the wrong direction.

Consent Boundaries Crossed

Here is an example of the confusion, and betrayal felt when boundaries are crossed and consent is disregarded:

A woman reported publicly in social media posts that she was touched inappropriately by a healer and leader in her community. This healer was also a musician who played the didgeridoo on the area of her vagina without asking for consent. He then had her lie down on a massage table for a Reiki treatment and placed her hand on her vagina area, putting his larger hand over hers. She told him that she felt uncomfortable doing this and that it felt too sexual for the healing session she was seeking. His response was to tell her that she was projecting her unhealed sexual wounding onto him and that she was overreacting—he was just doing healing work on her. This woman told him she disagreed, but continued the session which felt awkward and not healing. During their conversation before the session he did an astrology reading and frequently characterized her as having powerful sexual energy that she needed to heal and empower herself with.

Some women like the above example have expressed that they felt assaulted by some men presenting themselves as healers. These violations often seem to stem from the healer not making sure the client is fully *informed* of the type of treatment to be provided in the session and what that treatment involves—as well as not having clear consent for that treatment. In some cases, like this report, it is clearly an unconsented detour or change in the expected activity that oversteps boundaries and deviates from expected treatments. It's also apparent that some healers like the one described above, have an agenda or are imposing their expectation or assessment over what the client has asked for, even after being told they aren't comfortable with the treatment being applied. Healers must only provide treatments that are within the client's boundaries of consent—even if they think more advanced treatments would be beneficial to the client. The client's feelings and ability to absorb and integrate the treatments being applied is what is most important—not the healer's need or desire to provide certain treatments.

Consent and Personal Sexual Energy

Healers should be aware of how their personal sexual energy is impacting a client and from which energy center (yogic: Chakra) they are connecting with. There is a difference in the quality and character of energy coming from different energy centers which will have an effect on the client's experience. Energy can be directed from the Heart, or Brow (3rd eye) or from the Sacral/Root sex energy centers. Sexual healers do well to monitor their energy and realize which energy centers are active and engaging with their client. For sexual energy to be beneficially utilized in a sexual healing session and not harm the client, it must be *consciously and consensually engaged and activated with the awareness and consent of the client.*

Consent and Presence

A higher level of awareness is needed to guard against unintendedly harming a client by not being fully present and slipping into letting personal agendas take over. If this happens the healer is enacting patterns of personal intimacy, or unconscious sex rituals, and loses perspective as a responsible steward. In so doing, the healer drops into participating in the session at a more personal level that can surreptitiously attempt to satisfy emotional-sexual desires or fantasies. If this loss of objectivity and right-relationship happens it leaves the client vulnerable to being harmed.

For a sexual healer, remaining within the boundaries of consent means to diligently monitor their sexual energy and its interaction with their client, and remain present to what is happening in the moment—avoiding checking-out or fantasizing or detouring into unconscious sexual patterns.

Informed Consent

Informed Consent[11] is a legal term that shows up in several major areas of life: legal, medical, psychotherapy and counseling, and with business or insurance liability contracts. It is used as a way of formally establishing that a client has been apprised of potential dangers or side-effects which may impact the outcome of their experience. Typically with informed consent, there is a written declaration, statement or form that is read and signed by the client stating that they have read, understand and consent to the information contained in the statement.

Sexual Healers don't always use the formal informed consent process however, the principle of *completely informing* a client of treatment procedures, their likely or possible consequences and any side-effects, is important to understand and include in their practice.

To establish a container of trust and confidence in a sexual healing session there needs to be *transparency, openness,* and *honesty.* Being completely informed of possible treatment options—what the proposed treatment method includes along with any likely physical, emotional, and energetic consequences or side-effects—promotes confidence that allows a client to feel safe enough to participate and receive the benefits of treatments.

Transparency lets the client relax into trusting the sexual healer's ability to guide the session in a way that feels safe while being aided to consciously and safely expand their edge, and release and integrate their shadow and heal their wounds. Considering that sexual abuse is an infringement of one's ability to have a choice in what is happening to them; informed consent supports the client's process of rehabilitating their damaged sense of autonomy.

An additional consideration of informed consent is the client's ability to be in a *clear and competent* mental and emotional state to be able to affirm their participation and consent to treatment. The very nature of sexual healing sessions places the client in an emotionally and psychologically vulnerable position. A client's choices are filtered through this vulnerability and will need to have enough time to be processed before coming to a clear and competent settled conclusion. Sexual Healers might feel they know what is best for their client but should be careful not to push a client into consent by not allowing enough time to process their decision completely.

The Client

It is completely possible that someone may not have been abused, or even know they were abused or remember that any abuse happened to them—and so not feel they need sexual healing. Not everyone has been sexually abused or assaulted and not all abuse survivors have debilitating symptoms—but many do. There are also many people who for one reason or another have issues regarding sex and their ability to enjoy sex who could benefit from sexual healing treatments.

People who are survivors of sexual abuse trauma come from all walks of life, races, cultures and social status. Sexual abuse is prevalent and ubiquitous in modern culture and occurs in a wide range of forms and behaviors, some of which are not readily recognized as abusive.

Recent U.S. Statistics:

- Researchers have found that 1 in 6 men have experienced abusive sexual experiences before age 18. And this is *probably a low estimate* since it doesn't include noncontact experiences, which can also have lasting negative effects.[12]
- One in four college women reports surviving rape or attempted rape at some point in their lifetime.[13]
- 1 in 5 girls and 1 in 20 boys are a victim of child sexual abuse. The prevalence of child sexual abuse is difficult to determine because it is often not reported; experts agree that the *incidence is far greater than what is reported* to authorities.[14]

Survivors of sexual abuse seeking sexual healing will have emotional and psychological symptoms that can include: frightening memories, depression, low self-esteem, compulsive fantasies, dissociation, low libido, and an inability to sustain emotional intimacy in relationships. Addressing and healing these conditions involves reconnecting and integrating disparate and fragmented emotions and revitalizing a healthy body-mind-emotion integration, reclaiming personal power and autonomy, divesting debilitating thoughts and judgments, as well as processing, clearing and releasing feelings of fear, anger, rage, hurt, and emotional pain associated with sexual and emotional trauma.

Someone seeking help with sexual healing has reached a point where the pain and stress of carrying the wounds of the abuse are too much to bear any longer—making working on what is causing their symptoms imperative. Sometimes survivors will seek help when they reach a more mature age, or after suddenly remembering the abuse, or when attacks of invading thoughts become overwhelming; or sometimes it takes finding or developing supportive relationships that let them feel they can now work with sexual healing.

Not everyone who has experienced sexual trauma is ready to—or should—work with a sexual healer. Sexual healing is not a quick *retail-fix* where healing is purchased like so much orange juice from a convenience store. In cases where there is severe emotional and psychological trauma, abuse survivors should seek the care of a qualified therapist or counselor until they feel ready to work with a sexual healer.

Some sexual healers are therapists, or come from training in psychology and licensed therapy and are able to handle more severe cases of trauma and emotional wounding. Survivors having a hard time coping with more difficult symptoms should consult with a therapist prior to working with a sexual healer.

The domain of sexual healing includes a broad spectrum of issues and symptoms which include concerns and challenges that go beyond recovery from the trauma of sexual abuse. These can include any way that a person's sexuality is impacted such as with symptoms of low self-esteem, body dysmorphia, feelings of unworthiness, shame or guilt, or problems with relating, receiving or experiencing and sustaining intimacy with a partner.

Women's Experience

Safety is a key element that has to be present in order for sexual healing to be achievable. Too many women have been subjected to misogynous attitudes and abusive behavior which makes them feel unsafe and results in the contracting and diminishing of their natural expression and experience of sexuality. Over long periods of time in this state, women can start to shut down—put their sexuality *on hold* in a state of sexual limbo. The pain they feel from the abuse they experience causes them to shut down emotionally, and become detached from their feelings.

Conscientiously observing the principle of *ahimsa* (harmlessness) creates an environment of trustworthiness where female clients feel safe and autonomous and can open to healing from sexual abuse. Women are five times more likely than men to be sexually abused,[15] so they are particularly vulnerable when working with male sexual healers. For a woman to feel empowered sexually and open to her heart's deepest depths *she must feel safe.* Sexual healers should be sure to provide a safe presence and interact in a way that engenders the client's trust.

Reasons Some Women Seek Sexual Healing

The primary reason why women seek sexual healing is to recover from sexual trauma and return to sexual empowerment and integration. Besides seeking to heal from sexual abuse trauma, at different stages or circumstances in a woman's life she may need a safe and experienced guide to help her explore her sensual nature and release inhibiting or contracting feelings or beliefs around intimacy, self-worth, and wellbeing.

Additional reasons a woman might seek sexual healing with a male sexual healer are:

- Many women in our culture don't feel *safe enough* to let their sexual expression be fully felt, and therefore don't receive sexual fulfillment on a deeply enriching level. Sessions provide an opportunity to experience the fullness of a woman's erotic energy without the encumbrances of emotional attachments or reciprocal expectations. She can relax and open to allowing herself to feel her sensual, erotic energy without constraint or concern for pleasing her partner. This has a profound therapeutic effect that allows a woman to reclaim her sexual fullness, sensual confidence, and unabashed erotic expression.

- For different reasons, some women are inexperienced with men or being with male erotic energy. Sexual healing sessions allow them to experiment and broaden their experience in a safe, adept, trustworthy container where expectations and boundaries are clear and respected.

- Women often do not receive sincere unconditionally loving touch and acceptance from the men in their life. Or, they may not have any man available to meet their needs of touch and appreciation with unconditional love, acceptance, and validation. Sexual healing sessions can give a woman the experience of being with a man who helps her meet her needs and nurtures her sensual empowerment and mind-body integration.

- Some women have chosen to be celibate for a period of time. These women may want to experience or experiment with male energy in a safe container—either while celibate or coming out of being celibate before beginning a relationship with a man. The fact that no reciprocal pleasuring is expected of them helps them to relax into feeling their erotic energy in the presence of the sexual healer's positive male energy and maintain their choice of sexual celibacy.

- A woman might not have been in a sexual relationship in a while and wants to reconnect with her erotic energy without the expectation for sex or reciprocal treatment. After a break-up or in-between relationships, a woman may want to receive positive male attention and stay connected with her sensual energy without jumping into another relationship to receive it.

When women receive restorative sexual healing sessions they are rejuvenated and better able to transcend challenges and limitations, and achieve fuller self-expression and live their life more fully. Qualified and capable sexual healers are an important resource for women to achieve their goals of healing, empowerment, autonomy, and freedom.

Women working with Female Sexual Healers

For some women who are sexual abuse survivors, it isn't possible for them to consider working with a male sexual healer. Many women are completely comfortable, if not desirable of, working with another women in sensual exercises and interactions. For some women, working with another woman is the only way they will begin to heal their sexual abuse wounds.

The purpose of the session is not to have sex, but to facilitate the client's ability to be connected to, feel, and express their sensual energy and clear any emotional-energetic blocks that arise. Women are very capable of doing that for each other—men are needed if a female client desires to work with cis-gendered male energy. Women have masculine energy, as men have feminine energy, and to the degree a female sexual healer is able to access it, they can provide a *'masculine energy'* presence with a female client.

* For people who identify as LGBTQ+, it is important that you feel comfortable with who you work with and that you experience the masculine/feminine energy combination which works best for you. Seek a sexual healer who understands and empathizes with your sexual perspective and who has enough experience and insight to be competent in stewarding a session.

Men's Experience

Men have their own needs for sexual healing and emotional integration. Like women, men have been sexually abused, physically harmed, frequently judged and emotionally wounded. Men also suffer other challenges and insecurities like erectile dysfunction and premature ejaculation, poor body image, and anxiety due to lack of experience or misconceptions regarding sex and relationships.

Men are bombarded with media messages that stereotype a woman's body, her beauty and her place in society. Men can be confused about what intimacy and sex are—conflating the two. The possibility of relating intimately with women can scare men into hiding their feelings, pull away, or behave immaturely. In addition, men are usually unaware of, or unfamiliar with, their inner feminine energy. Men can greatly benefit from a safe, adept female sexual healer who can awaken and guide them to a relationship with their inner feminine, and help them heal their relationship with women.

Many men are seeking the *divine feminine* to be present in their life through a deeper, chthonic spirituality initiating them into spiritual-sexual integration. When a female practitioner leads a sexual healing session for a man she can greatly affect his psyche and help him to engage with women with a new level of respect and appreciation.

For men to experience optimum sexual expression and integration it is essential that they have an awareness and understanding of sexual energy, cultivate an integrated heart-genital connection, slow down their sexual impulses, and break unconscious sexual patterns while expanding their ability to experience prolonged pleasure. By learning to be consciously aware of sexual energy and be adept at modulating, circulating, and flowing with it, a man can realize his optimal sexual capabilities and increase his spiritual connection with sex to become a more present and heart-centered lover. Men can get the education and healing experience they need to accomplish all of this in sexual healing or erotic enrichment sessions.

What Clients Should Know

Clients seeking sexual healing are looking for someone capable of deep empathy and adept at creating and maintaining the therapeutic container for their healing process. Choosing a sexual healer is in some ways like choosing any healthcare practitioner who assess emotional and physical wellbeing and who interacts with the body. Competency, training, trust, and compatibility are important considerations. Above all, potential clients want to feel safe.

Establishing a rapport of trust and safety involves transparency and clarity. Clients are willing to trust someone they don't know very well to help them experience their growth-edge and heal their abuse wounds if they understand and agree with treatment boundaries and are informed of the potential side-effects and outcomes possible from such treatments.

At a basic level, a potential client will want to know the sexual healer's training, education, and experience, as well as what type of session is being offered and what activities are to be included and excluded in the session. They will want to know how sexual healing sessions can benefit them and why a type of treatment is appropriate for their condition and how it will help them recover or find relief.

To find out if a sexual healer is the right fit, the client may also want to know about the healer's spiritual perspective or practice and what continuing education and training they've received.

Before having a session with a sexual healer an in-person, phone, or webcam interview is important to aid in determining if the healer is the right fit for the client. During this interview, it's important to have a candid discussion that answers the client's questions and clarifies their intention for the session.

Potential clients should watch out for promises of miraculous results using invasive treatments like "yoni healing" or "g-spot massage" offered with little consideration of the consequences associated with processing sexual abuse trauma. Without adequate preparation and emotional support, an abuse survivor can be further traumatized.

One of the potentials for harming clients is a "retail mindset" by the practitioner, client or both principals. Sexual healing is not a *buy it off the shelf product* or a quick-fix solution. It is a service that is best administered with long-term expectations that allow the establishment of a relationship of trust and adequate time for releasing and integrating complex emotions from abuse wounds. No benefit is received—and potentially great harm can be experienced— if the healer misrepresents their capabilities, treatment effectiveness or session expectations.

Red Flags to Watch Out For

When choosing a sexual healer—and afterward as their client—there are some things to watch out for that are red flags of warning and alert.

- **Healer is too familiar.** Interactions feel inappropriately "close" or at a level of intimacy beyond professional.

  Caring about clients' welfare and progress produces endearment over time, however, there should always be a professional boundary which provides objectivity and supports a healthy *healing alliance* relationship. If the relationship is allowed to slip into becoming more personal than professional it can create a situation where boundaries feel vague or confusing, and which can be easily crossed.

  It might also be an indication that the sexual healer is using their clients for a personal relationship or vicarious sexual fulfillment and would, therefore, contaminate sessions with their personal issues and projections. Remedying this may be as simple as sharing your feelings and asking for clarity and professionalism with interactions. If this doesn't restore an appropriate healing alliance relationship the client should look for a different healer.

- **Healer isn't explicit and transparent about treatments.** Healers should be able to thoroughly discuss treatments and activities to be included in sessions, and not withhold significant details from clients that get sprung on them during a session. A sexual healer should be able to explain why a certain treatment is being recommended, what the outcomes are likely to be, and what the possible side-effects, down-side, or limitations such a treatment could have.

- **Healer wants to get naked with you in sessions.** This is an obvious tip that the healer is ungrounded and has a personal agenda they are acting out in the treatments they provide to clients. Sexual healing treatments do not normally require the healer to be unclothed to facilitate them. Client nudity or partial nudity should be optional and being nude should be inappropriate for the healer. In some cases where client and healer have established rapport and trust over several sessions, the client might choose to be unclothed—but there is seldom a good reason for a healer to be nude with a client. That being said, one reason a sexual healer might be nude with a client is when the client requests it to feel *equally exposed and vulnerable.* If this is the case, the sexual healer will want to cover the potential unwanted effects mentioned here with the client during consent discussions.

In the context and environment of private sexual healing sessions, mutual nudity makes a subliminal statement that the interactions in the session are more sexual and personal instead of therapeutic or healing. If both the client and healer are nude together in a session, it elicits physiological and psychological responses which activate unconscious, personal sex behavior.

- **Healer crosses boundaries of consented treatments and activities.** Whenever a client feels their boundaries have been crossed, they should immediately speak up and halt session activities and ask the healer for an explanation.

There may be times when inadvertent and innocent mistakes are made—however, more than one occurrence means either the healer isn't paying attention, doesn't care, or has ulterior motives. Any of these occurrences repeated more than once should halt the treatment and potentially disqualify them from further interaction with the client.

Survivors of abuse should not be further abused because of a healer's recklessness or callousness. When that kind of mistake is made it's a strong indication that the session needs to slow down or pause, and possibly stop. Much more awareness and presence must be established before going further—and clients will want to evaluate whether or not to continue working with the healer.

- **Healer provides a different treatment than what was discussed.** Clients report feeling shocked and "frozen" when their healer did something they had not discussed beforehand; which was completely different from what they said they would provide. Some felt they needed to go along with the undisclosed treatments even when they weren't comfortable with them because they were afraid to speak up. They felt they had to "let him do it" so that "maybe he will stop or move on to what he said he would do."

If this happens to you and you can speak up—do so immediately and confront the healer—or get up and leave the session, call someone to pick you up and stay with you until you feel safe again. Don't tolerate misleading or manipulative healers and report their behavior to whoever referred you to them.

Diminished Capacity Considerations:

Diminished capacity is when someone is not able to make decisions or take actions that are in their best interest and safety due to being in a state of mind, health condition, environment, or under a substance's influence. Being sleep deprived, sick, grieving, insecure, or under the influence of anything that creates diminished capacity should be a red flag warning to not have a sexual healing session or to stop one that has begun.

Never consent to a sexual healing session when inebriated or high, and don't go into a sexual healing session under the influence of anything which will affect your capacity to report/indicate/voice any change in your consent of session treatments. If for any reason during a session the client is no longer in consent, they need to be able to express the changed state of their truth. The sexual healer should welcome this input and make an immediate adjustment to the session, pausing to discuss the arisen feelings and reestablish consent for further treatment or end the session.

Somatic Trance / Tantric Thrall

In sexual healing sessions, many treatments are designed to relax the body and drop emotional/physical armoring or clenching to allow activated erotic energy to clear away blockages and encourage energy flow. Somatic trance is a trance-like state that massage clients are familiar with. It happens when a client becomes extremely relaxed to the point of "drifting off" mentally—sometimes falling asleep during a massage.

Besides relaxing the body, sexual healing treatments frequently add pleasuring the body's erogenous areas to activate and build erotic energy to flow throughout the client's energy matrix. This produces a trance-like effect known as "Tantric Thrall" which puts the subject in a state of mind that is under the influence of the pleasure being experienced to the point of not being fully in control and not mindfully present to what is being done. Tantric Thrall produces mild to severe states of dissociation which puts the subject in a diminished capacity to control their experience or object to what is happening.

What can clients do about it?

Clients in sexual healing sessions should try to remain present to what is happening and not "check-out." Attention should be focused on the sensations felt in the present moment, going deeper into the sensation being experienced. Dissociation is a common symptom that survivors of sexual abuse have. If a client is having difficulties remaining present when experiencing pleasure, the sexual healer should use introductory exercises or treatments that will gently and slowly help the client remain present and become more embodied in the experience.

A great amount of trust is placed on sexual healers by their clients due to the somatic trance and Tantric thrall phenomena which can happen with sexual healing treatments. Make sure your sexual healer has demonstrated respect for your state of mind, emotions, and consent in pre-session interviews or intake conversations—and question or raise objections if they are not mindful and respectful of your autonomy and safety. Referrals are a good indicator of trustworthiness, and initial sessions should take things slowly and incrementally so that a client feels confident in their healer's integrity and respect for their wellbeing.

If a client feels they are beginning to slip into a dissociative state during a session—say something to the healer. They should have already been aware of your drifting (noticing the signs of "checking out"—spacing out or languishing attention, non-responsive to prompts or inquiry, a disconnect in emotional or physical response, abrupt mood shift, depression, or emotional outburst not associated with present interactions) and should pause the session to re-establish presence and reconnect with what is happening and allow for processing of the emotions that have come up.

Relaxing, letting go, surrendering, or releasing the mind's dominance is not the same as dissociation. Staying present during session treatments takes the client deeper into what is happening by feeling more and being more aware of the sensations experienced. Checking out takes the client somewhere else that is away from what is happening—off into another time, memory, or fantasy that is not connected to the experience in the session. There's a big difference between being caught up in the pleasure of what may be happening and checking out into dissociative states. Sexual healers should know how to spot this and know what to do to bring someone back to the Now moment and help them process what they've experienced.

After some sessions have transpired, client and healer will have established a rapport that recognizes when the client is heading towards *checking-out* and can readily be handled. The client can eventually develop a better awareness of when the onset of a dissociative state begins (common thoughts or feelings just prior to onset) and take measures to remain present with the experience (breathing, focused attention, embodiment awareness). Treatments can/should also include helping the client with methods of self-care and self-treatment to mitigate dissociative onset outside of sexual healing sessions (i.e. when with their partner or when triggered in a dating/socializing setting).

Clients might also feel *a little off*—a sense of "floating"—after a sexual healing session. This might impact their ability to drive and safely return home. After a session, the sexual healer should make sure their client is able to function adequately and is able to get to their destination. Clients should never drive or walk alone if they feel ungrounded or dissociative. They should wait at the healer's location or call a friend or taxi/Uber to be transported safely.

Stages of the Sexual Healing Process

Sexual healing is a process of reclaiming oneself and reconnecting psychological and emotional elements of the psyche that have been fragmented, suppressed, denied, unrecognized or ignored due to wounds of sexual abuse, assault, and emotional trauma.

Some traumatized people have only a vague awareness of something happening to them in the past. They may avoid looking at it too closely because of the fear and pain associated with it. If sexual abuse survivors are aware of having been abused they usually don't want to think or talk about it. Instead, they try to stuff their feelings into a metaphorical jail cell *out-of-sight* and not deal with them.

Inwardly, abuse survivors often feel detached from feeling deep emotion and connection. Abuse survivors can also feel disconnected from the sensations of their body—stuck *in their head* with a disembodied awareness of experience. Recalling memories that reveal abuse produces a lot of anxiety and fear and will affect interactions with others, especially those who the survivor is close to.

There are several aspects to the process of sexual healing that often come in stages which lead into each other. These stages or phases of sexual healing-recovery outline a *possible progression of* steps sexual abuse survivors might experience while seeking and getting help. The following is a progression of stages derived from my experience with my clients which might or might not be experienced by other sexual abuse survivors in their unique case:

Victim – Survivor

Victimhood could be defined as *the state of being taken advantage of or harmed by another, especially in a crime or accident. The state of having suffered as a result of someone else's actions.*

When sexual abuse trauma occurs there is a wound created by the psychological and emotional overwhelm of the experience. In some cases, disassociation occurs, with some people feeling disembodied and viewing the abuse from floating above it or leaving the location to *remote-view* elsewhere. Such experiences can be suppressed, shut down and stuffed into the dark corners of the psyche.

Suppressed feelings from abuse or trauma don't stay nicely tucked away. Eventually, dreams, memories, flashbacks or visions of the abuse start to break through into conscious awareness. Survivors experiencing memories or flashbacks that are too much to handle, or too hard to figure out by themselves often see a therapist or counselor for help.

For a sexual trauma survivor, sometimes just acknowledging the abuse is a tremendous accomplishment. What to do next can be daunting and difficult to figure out. There can be many competing concerns and fears which are emotionally and energetically immobilizing and yet, remaining silent can also be excruciating.

Fear

At some point, a survivor may realize that their deep pain and overwhelming emotions are too much to handle alone. It can feel like a brooding, impending catastrophe that seems to have a will of its own—who wants to reveal itself and be dealt with.

Fear inspires questions like "What will happen if I let this out?"

"If this pain gets uncorked will it wreak havoc on my life?"

"Is it worth it—the toll of going through emotional turmoil and feeling exposed and vulnerable?"

At this stage, previously suppressed and ignored feelings about the abuse can surface to be released and these can contain a lot of fear. It can make a survivor feel like their world is being turned upside down. Fear can be a huge block to further progress in healing.

For a survivor to move beyond fear, it must become more important to heal than it is to avoid their feelings. Anything that stretches a comfort zone or addresses fears or wounds will feel scary. Fear can become an ally and show us where to look for more complete healing. Once a survivor decides to get sexual healing, it's up to the sexual healer to provide a container that feels safe for an abuse survivor to open up and work with their fears, and begin healing.

Frustration to Determination

Another stage of the process of sexual healing is feeling the frustration of being caught between a hard place and a rock. There can be an inner imperative to take steps to stop feeling terrible, worthless, and ashamed, which is opposed by a paralyzing fear of accepting and dealing with all of it—that produces frustration.

If a survivor is in a relationship, their inner turmoil and frustration will likely have an impact on the relationship's intimacy and sexual fulfillment. The weight of all of this emotional pain and frustration can be too much; resulting in alcohol or drug abuse, eating disorders, or sexually acting out. Abuse survivors can try to stuff their emotions and hope they will just go away—or sometimes they will give up and assume that they will just have to be miserable.

For those who try to get past their frustration and inner turmoil in hopes of finding answers and feeling better, a determination can emerge. These survivors can no longer avoid or ignore their condition or the haunting knowledge that invades their thoughts and relationships. Determined to succeed, they renew their search for answers and will try alternative therapies and self-help solutions or traditional medicine treatments hoping these will provide relief.

Despair to Courage

If after trying self-help solutions or traditional treatments, these prove ineffective or short-lived, a return of symptoms and emotional upheaval and depression is possible. Once again, the abuse survivor can be faced with the choice to give up or to press forward to find real and lasting solutions. If they find the courage to continue, often this renewed determination will lead them eventually to a healer they can work with who is trained and has experience with sexual healing.

Most people don't know about sexual healing, let alone know anyone who is a sexual healer. The dilemma is like having a medical condition that requires a specialist and not knowing that such a specialty exists—or where to find a specialist even if they knew they needed one. So, the first hurdle is knowing about sexual healing. The second one is finding a competent sexual healer to work with. Hopefully, the information in this book will help in accomplishing both objectives.

A survivor is next faced with the reality that their condition is treatable and someone is available to help them heal. The realization of this possibility can again prompt fears of "opening up a can of worms." It takes a great deal of courage to persevere to this point and determinedly follow through and begin sessions with a sexual healer.

For a long time, the abuse survivor has held onto emotional and psychological wounds and some survivors may wonder how will the healing process affect them, how will they change?

Crossroads and Success

When an abuse survivor commits to working with a sexual healer or other practitioner specializing in sexual healing, a new set of circumstances, reactions, and emotions are unleashed.

Initially, having a specialist who understands and can offer solutions and a path forward is a huge relief. However, the work is just beginning and there will be more challenges that surface throughout the process of healing. When treatments begin, there can be a release of pent-up emotion—activated by the simplest or slightest addressing of their condition.

A survivor's ability to withstand the emotional and psychological toll that the healing process can exact will be a significant factor in their relief and recovery. At any time throughout their healing process, trauma wounds can be triggered and have a profound impact on a survivor's state of mind and emotional balance. Sometimes this is too much for a client to handle and they will stop a session or end further treatment.

It is the sexual healer's responsibility to steward sessions and implement treatments that don't give a client more than they can handle. However, in some cases, even the most careful and gentle implementation can trigger a client's reaction. Once again, a survivor's determination and courage to continue the healing process is essential to getting relief and making progress in recovering and moving forward.

A crossroads is reached when the discomfort resulting from the emotional and psychological pain that turns up during sessions is weighed against the consequences of stopping and living with the suffering. Survivors can feel confused and anxious, which is amplified by the knowledge there is a path leading to healing but which feels too much to bear at present. In some cases, clients who stop sexual healing sessions come back after a period of time of allowing their emotions and fears to settle.

Each person is different and will have a different response, pace of realization, and rate of progress with healing. Relief and recovery will be reached with successive treatments and sessions. Those who persevere with their healing must sustain their ability to handle the revelations of their wounds and the emotions that come up in their healing process.

What Does Successfully Healed Look Like?

Successful healing is reached when a survivor's memories or activated emotions are no longer overwhelming or debilitating and no longer create emotional sabotage or derailment and the survivor is able to return to a sense of wholeness and wellbeing. It is a success when they can have relationships without their trauma wounds intervening and causing undue stress or diminishing their ability to sustain intimacy. It is a success when a survivor is able to feel sensual and have sex without shame and feel an empowered autonomy over their body and what happens to them.

Finding a Sexual Healer who is the Right Fit

It may be a challenge to find a sexual healer to work with until sexual healing becomes more widely accepted and approved as an alternative healing modality.

You could ask your friends about sexual healing—you might be surprised to find out they have worked with a healer before and possibly, they would be willing to share with you about their experience. Sexual healing is very personal and confidential, often clients don't talk about it very much or share their process with other people very openly. If someone you know and trust has shared their experience of sexual healing with you, you could ask them for a referral with the healer they worked with.

Another way to find a sexual healer is to do a search online for "sexual healing," "Tantric healing," or "Tantric massage." You could also attend a local Tantra group and ask for referrals. I've included in the Appendix of this book a list of schools that certify sexual healers that you can contact for referrals. If you are under the care of a therapist you could ask them if they know of any sexual healers and possibly be referred by them.

Alternatively, you could approach a trusted and qualified bodyworker, e.g. Myofascial Release Therapist, or a massage therapist, or a Physical Therapist and if necessary, sign a release granting permission for treatments to 'private areas' of the body (including if necessary invasive treatments such as *Internal Pelvic Release.*)

Finding the right sexual healer for *you* can be a process that takes some time. Not all practitioners are the same or offer the same treatments. A good fit for one person may not be a good fit for another person. Sexual healers realize that not everyone will be a good fit as a client and won't be offended if a potential client chooses to not work with them. Set up an in-person interview, or at least a Skype or phone conversation, to have your questions answered and to see if both client and healer are a good fit for working together.

Healing Takes Time

Survivors of sexual abuse and assault need to know that there are usually no quick fixes; no miracle cures or magic wands that can be waved to take away the emotional pain, guilt, or shame, associated with their wounds. Clients need to be willing to invest the time it takes for their unique process of healing to find fruition.

Sexual healing and recovery are not likely to happen after one, or even a few sessions. Plan on allowing for all the time you need to complete the healing process without unrealistic expectations. The more openness, energy and focus a survivor is able to devote to their healing and transformation the more effective and faster their healing process will be.

There will also be relapses in reoccurrences of symptoms which may get triggered situationally, or arise spontaneously after having been addressed in previous treatments and sessions—with clients expecting they were complete with them. Clients will often need "refresher" sessions and require a deeper look at, and a redressing of some issues they thought were healed. This is not unusual or abnormal and should be accepted as part of the process of healing and not a setback or regression.

The Best You Can Hope For

Completing the healing process won't erase the memories of the abuse or trauma. However, sexual healing *is* capable of providing relief by lessening the frequency and impact of thoughts or memories so they won't be debilitative or overwhelming. Sexual healing can enable survivors to feel integrated and whole again and regain their sense of sexual empowerment and personal autonomy and feel capable of working with their emotions and sustain intimate relationships.

The best situation a survivor of sexual trauma can hope for is to no longer be emotionally fragmented, derailed, or set back due to invasive thoughts or feelings that come from their trauma. Survivors will always have the acknowledgment of the trauma they experienced and know the facts about what happened. With sexual healing, success is defined as no longer being controlled or compelled by those memories, thoughts, or feelings—to the point that they no longer sabotage or derail relationships or create personal inner turmoil. They may not be able to forget what happened, but they can move forward as integrated and whole people who are empowered and no longer debilitated by their experience.

Client Checklist for Safe Sexual Healing

Survivors of sexual abuse can be confident that there is effective help available and that they can achieve a sense of wholeness and wellbeing if they are prepared for the process they must go through to get there. It's like needing serious medical treatment to recover from an accident—it will be a process that can include some pain and discomfort, but if the treatment is not completed the symptoms will continue and the survivor will continue to suffer from their condition.

Breakthroughs can happen quickly, but it takes time to integrate the changes at a mental, emotional, and somatic level. After-care is as important as what happens during sexual healing sessions with the sexual healer. Some of the items in the following list are about what can be done in follow-up to healing sessions to help integrate the results.

This checklist isn't *everything* that is needed to be considered and not all of these suggestions will apply to everyone—but it's a good start. Use good sense and your gut intuition during the entire process and when in doubt—ask. Survivors must be able to speak up and be their own best advocate, which can be difficult to do when feeling broken or emotionally destitute. A good sexual healer will also be a strong advocate who vigilantly keeps their client on track and making progress toward healing.

1. Are you ready?

Emotionally & Energetically

There will be an emotional and energetic cost that will affect your life. The process of discovering, identifying, releasing and healing from sexual abuse can feel like your world is being turned upside down. Your sexual healer will help you deal with the emotions that are unleashed, but you must be prepared to experience emotional discomfort and spend time with self-care outside of the sessions. Take stock of your circumstances and prepare yourself to go through what may be a very difficult process. It's important to have support besides your healer (see below).

Physical

Your body is a repository for emotional memory and will benefit from complementary treatments in addition to sexual healing sessions. Optimum physical health will help you feel stronger emotionally and go through the healing process with more energy. See if you can improve your diet, exercise, and sleep routines so you will have enough energy reserves to continue with your healing program.

Time

Not only do you need time to have healing sessions, but you must also give yourself adequate time to process and integrate the effects of what your healing process reveals or triggers. Realize that you'll likely need space in your schedule to reflect upon the emotions and realizations that are discovered in your healing sessions. Also, there will likely be exercises or practices to be done at home; given to you by your healer that will aid you with your healing. Give yourself the time you need to do these follow-up exercises, meditations, and activities.

Cost

There can be a significant cost involved to complete a program of healing which could take several months or more. Each client is different, so the time it takes and the number of sessions needed to complete the healing process is unknown until the goal of returning to wholeness and empowered wellbeing is reached. What is most important is that you find a sexual healer you can work with and feel confident in, and budget your expenses to accommodate the cost.

2.   Finding a sexual healer you feel good about.

It's important to interview a potential sexual healer to make sure you feel they are "a good fit" and you feel comfortable opening up to them. Even though you may have an impacted or diminished sense of trust in others due to surviving sexual trauma, your gut feeling is still your best indicator of who is best for you to work with. If you have reached the point where sexual healing is imperative for you, then trust in your due diligence, and let your intuition lead you to the right person to work with.

Ask the potential sexual healer where they were trained and by whom, as well as how many years of experience they have. Ask if they have any references from clients that they can share with you (these might not be available due to the highly confidential nature of sexual healing). At the very least they should have testimonials to share with you. If they belong to an affiliate association you can check to see if they are in good standing.

Due to the burgeoning nature of sexual healing and its semi-illicitness in many areas of the world, sexual healers have had to operate in the shadows of society to provide their services. This is gradually changing with more public awareness and support, but until it is completely out in the open and accepted, complete transparency may be difficult to come by. Do your best to find out the sexual healer's qualifications, experience, and reputation, and after an interview or consultation trust your intuition.

3. Have a support system.

Personal

Establish a practice of working with your emotions and the revealing insights and thought patterns that are associated with your trauma wounds. Doing things like meditation, journaling, and personal nurturing (hot soaks, contemplative walks, body pampering, creative outlets) are important to arrange and make time for.

Buddy System

In addition to your healer, it's important to have a buddy system with at least one person who knows what you're going through and will be a resource of unconditional support. Choose someone close to you to be your confidant who is good at listening and won't judge you. Have regular *"shares"* with this person throughout your healing process.

Community

If possible, seek out others who have also gone through sexual healing (local Meetup group, 12 step group, Tantra group, or the like). They can provide a safety net in the event that you need additional support, or if your personal confidant is not available.

4. Get additional professional support.

Therapist – Counselor

It is important that any sexual abuse survivor be confident in their ability to handle and process the strong emotions associated with sexual healing. If there's any doubt or reservation about that, then they should first work with a therapist or counselor and become emotionally capable before proceeding with sexual healing.

For some clients, it's also a good idea to continue to work with a therapist or counselor while working with a sexual healer. Make sure anyone you work with will be supportive of your decision to work with a sexual healer.

Doctor – Alternative Healer – Shaman

Additional healing resources are sometimes necessary especially when physical health issues are present. Consult with your doctor or another qualified healer to make sure you are not neglecting or omitting important medical treatments where these apply. Let your sexual healer know of any medications with side-effects that may influence your state of mind or emotions during sessions.

Alternative Healers or Shamans can provide healing resources on other levels that the physicians of traditional medicine don't provide. It may be beneficial to consult with an alternative healer or shaman to receive non-traditional therapies that could be effective in helping your healing process (e.g. Acupuncture, Reiki, or Myofascial Release Therapy).

Spiritual Advisor

You will feel better and make quicker progress if you also consider the spiritual element of your healing process. Consult with a spiritual advisor to get support and/or *spiritual healing* while you go through your sexual healing program.

5. Check in with your support ally

Important pre-and-post session care is to check in with someone who knows what you're going through, and knows what you're doing, and let them know when and where you are having sessions. This is a safety step, not out of distrust of your healer (you should only work with someone you trust completely) it is in consideration of possible sudden emotional shifts that can result from your sexual healing sessions. It's possible to become disoriented or suddenly fall into bouts of despair or depression due to mood swings caused by uncovering disturbing memories or from processing strong emotions. Checking-in, especially after sessions, will help you feel safe and supported regardless of whether or not you have a sudden shift in your state of being.

You should never leave a healing session in a psychologically fragmented state of shock. Your sexual healer should be able to accommodate that circumstance should it happen and remain with you until you feel grounded, competent and able to leave or until your buddy support arrives.

6. Keep a journal.

Writing to yourself about your feelings, memories, and breakthroughs will help you process and learn from them. Writing out your stream of thought, or writing things down so you can remember them, are two ways that journaling can help. The act of writing combines a kinesthetic, mental, and emotional process which can effectively relieve emotional inflammation and facilitate psychological integration and the release of trauma.

A journal is just for your eyes only. Writing out your feelings and re-reading them again later can provide a different perspective and new insight. Journaling about your discoveries and accomplishments helps to mark progress and appreciate the deepening awareness you are discovering about yourself.

7. Take care of yourself.

Time for integration

As mentioned above, it is important to give yourself time for integrating and processing the feelings that come up and the insights revealed in your sessions. Allow enough space between sessions so you can process and integrate things to a satisfactory extent before taking on another session.

Physical and energetic integration is also important and is achieved through rest and de-stressing practices. Make time for when you are not processing but are just recharging your batteries and resting. This also means taking every opportunity throughout the day to release stress, tension, and anxiety. Maintain a practice of calming and relaxing yourself, and listen to your body's need for rest and sleep.

Sleep

Related to the above is to have enough, and good sleep. This is important for your mind, energy, and body to recuperate, balance, and recharge. You need to reach the deep REM state of sleep several times a night. If you are getting up a lot, or can't get to sleep early enough, you are likely not getting the rest your body and mind require to function optimally.

Exercise

Moving your body, stretching, and exercising your muscles will help move the impacted energy and shake up embedded patterns stored somatically in the body. This will help speed and facilitate your healing.

Bodywork

As mentioned previously, bodywork is beneficial for helping to move impacted energy and clearing your body of embedded psychosomatic energy knots resulting from emotional trauma. Try to arrange for regular bodywork treatments to help with releasing what sexual healing sessions will activate, stimulate, or trigger.

Tantric Healing Sessions

For those who have become aware of, and are learning about the ancient spiritual-sexual-science called "Tantra," another place where there can be an exposure to harm is during Tantra events, workshops, or in "Tantric healing" sessions. Be careful when attending and participating in Tantra workshops or in Tantric healing sessions with teachers or facilitators. There have been several sexual assault and rape allegations made against some of the most prominent Tantra schools and their leaders/teachers/healers. [16]

"Tantra" (Neo-Tantra)

The practice of Tantra in the West (neo-Tantra) includes many different expressions and different understandings of what Tantra is. The word *Tantra* seems to have become a catch-all term for all things that effect, improve, expand, enhance, educate, initiate, inspire, and heal, with sexual energy, and are about spiritual sexuality and enhanced sexual expression.

Consequently, Tantra healing sessions can be very open-ended and free-flowing, or they can also be focused on one or a few aspects of understanding and experiencing sexual energy. The term *Tantric healing* can be used as a synonym for sexual healing even though there may be little *Tantra*—as it is traditionally known—being practiced.

To me, the term has validity in that it signifies a level of understanding of sexual energy that is relevant and important to the sexual healing process. In addition to having a familiarity and an understanding of sexual energy, Tantric sexual healers should have at least a basic knowledge and understanding of human physiology and the psychological impact that sexual healing can have on clients.

If you are considering having Tantric Healing sessions with someone, the same concerns and consent considerations will apply as they would with a sexual healer. At the very least, discuss what activities the session will include, as well as activity boundaries and who is doing what to whom—and reach a consensual agreement.

Making Tantra and Sexual Healing Workshops Safe

There are many Tantra training schools and workshops offering participants an enhanced understanding and experience with sexual energy. In these workshops, the principles of sexual healing are often included because clearing blocks to personal sexual experience are part of sexual empowerment and autonomy. However, an unintended result of this has been to encourage some unqualified people to become sexual healers for others without much in-depth training.

The information gained in Tantra workshops and training can be good for an individual to begin their *personal process* of self-discovery and sexual healing but it is often not comprehensive enough to be safely used to help someone else. Those who practice Tantra, especially those just beginning their Tantric education, do well to get more comprehensive training and take the time necessary to process and understand their own sexual abuse trauma issues with help from qualified teachers and coaches before attempting to become sexual healers for other people.

Without adequate planning and safeguards in place, one area where there is the opportunity for unintended harm to participants is in Tantra workshops. These types of workshops can expose participants to shadow aspects of their psyche and call up sexual abuse trauma wounds. This is particularly important when workshop participation includes invasive, internal work (penetration of the vagina or anus— e.g. internal pelvic release, female ejaculation, and prostate work or other pelvic integration procedures) without adequate preparation, participants are likely to be triggered and suffer emotional harm.

Workshop facilitators are responsible for the wellbeing and safety of their workshop participants. Facilitators should be aware of how the sequence of their workshop modules and their emotional impact contributes to a participant's ability to absorb and integrate the material being presented. Leading unprepared and vulnerable participants into experiences that can cause emotional harm or psychological shock is reckless, naïve, irresponsible, and harmful to the participants.

Facilitators who don't realize the impact an activity could have, or know how to handle adverse reactions to treatments or activities, or don't think there is a possibility of harm happening, are responsible for any harm that occurs from their unpreparedness. Such was the case with a well-meaning *goddess retreat* that failed to realize the impact that the sequence of modules on deep shadow work, Tantra, and sexual healing would have on their participants.

By the fifth day of seven, three women had to leave; one went to the hospital seeking medical care for her anxiety, another sought help from a therapist, and the third woman was helped by her family's support—who threatened legal action. None of the volunteers staffing the event were trained to respond to emotional fragmentation or shock, and no one had considered the emotional triggers that might occur given the limited integration time in the schedule—in addition there was no 'workshop buddy' safety net in place to detect a problem before it was too late.

To create a safe workshop experience, some basic precautions will go a long way to ensure participants are adequately protected:

- Adequate staffing of trained assistants familiar with helping people process and integrate difficult emotions and triggered trauma wounds.
- Facilitator and assistants trained in spotting and handling, acute stress reaction, anxiety, psychological trauma, and emotional fragmentation.
- Allow adequate time during the workshop for processing and integration with support—especially when invasive techniques are being taught
- Awareness of, and planning for the psychological impact of the workshop and the impact that the workshop module sequence is likely to produce.
- Due consideration for emotional and energetic safety for participants (from voyeur or "leech" energy) while they are vulnerable/exposed when doing workshop exercises or training.
- Application screening with questions such as the following:

Are you under the care of a physician or therapist, and are you on any psychiatric medications?

Who/what is your backup safety net should you need additional support during or after the workshop?

- Use of a workshop "buddy system" during the event, with frequent check-ins.

Signs of acute stress, anxiety, and psychological shock can include any of the following: [17, 18, 19]

- A sense of numbing, detachment, or absence of emotional responsiveness.
- A reduction in awareness of his or her surroundings (e.g., being in a daze).
- Dissociative amnesia (i.e., inability to recall an important aspect of the trauma).
- Persistent re-experiencing of the traumatic occurrence in the form of recurrent images, thoughts, dreams, illusions, flashback episodes, or a sense of reliving the experience.
- Distress on exposure to reminders of the traumatic event.
- Anger, irritability, or mood swings.
- Confusion or difficulty concentrating.
- Feeling overwhelmed or emotionally fragmented.
- Tension, cramping, tingling, "pins and needles" feeling, shortness of breath, anxiety, nervousness, or a sense of doom.

While Tantra workshops can offer valuable experiences, caution on the part of the organizers and facilitators should be exercised so participants can benefit without unintentionally being harmed in the process.

Tantra workshops and HPV

Another safety exposure during workshops that use a Tantra "puja" type of activity—where partners rotate around a circle from one station to the next performing various sensual energy exercises and intimate interactions with each person. Group work and activities like this can expose participants to possible communicable infections if precautions are not made.

In Tantra workshops and pujas, some activities can involve sensual touch—and for some activities wardrobe outfits with minimal covering provide for a skin to skin contact of the genital area (e.g. sitting "Yab-Yum" on the lap of a participant) which invites possible exposure to HPV transmission. Workshop facilitators should discuss safer sex and HPV information with the group and ask participants to maintain a barrier between themselves and another participant's genital area when activities warrant it.

Don't Give Up

A survivor of sexual abuse or trauma has a daunting journey to undertake to heal and reach wholeness again. It can be challenging and requires determination and persistence but returns great rewards when accomplished. Despite the many challenges facing sexual trauma survivors, there is hope. Capable, understanding and safe sexual healers are ready to help you to process and release the trauma wounds you carry and return to a sense of safety and well-being, autonomy, and empowerment. It takes great courage and determination to take on and complete your healing process—and with qualified healing facilitators, you can achieve the healing you seek.

The Healer

Sexual Healers help their clients to address their sexual trauma and unresolved emotional issues that impact sexual experience in order to heal and achieve a sense of wellbeing and wholeness again. Sexual healers who serve women do so to be part of their healing solution and not to become a perpetrator of further sexual abuse. Male sexual healers have an incredible opportunity to align with a higher expression of masculinity—one that is unconditionally loving and accepting and that supports their client's empowerment by making sure they protect the safety and integrity of the healing session.

The sexual healer works with a client's sexual energy to free it from the hold of past trauma, cultural stereotypes, and unconscious beliefs that inhibit, contract, or suppress sexual experience and a fluent body–mind–emotion integration. A sexual healer is in the service of *entelechy* —the evolutionary urge to advance, grow, mature, heal or better oneself—and bears great responsibility for their client's welfare and experience while working with them.

Sexual healers can come from many different counseling, coaching, and healing modalities. They can be any personal improvement or healing provider who addresses issues around intimacy, touch, or emotional trauma occurring from sexual abuse or which effects sexual experience.

Sexual healers are known by many different terms—in recent years a new professional designation of "sexologist" or sexological bodyworker has been introduced, and in neo-Tantra circles the terms "Daka" (male sexual healer) or "Dakini" (female sexual healer) are prevalent. Each of these, and many others can have their own methodology and facilitation of sexual healing sessions.

If you feel called to be a sexual healer, thank you. As a healer in service to another's transformation at the most intimate and vulnerable levels of being you are being asked to provide your utmost in presence, stewardship, and integrity. What follows are basic areas where sexual healers should be proficient in understanding and implementing with their clients—the most important of which is Consent.

Consent

Nothing is more important to the sexual healer than a client's active and current consent with the activities and treatments of a healing session. The following are some important points about consent that a sexual healer will want to make sure they are abiding by, and are responsive to while facilitating session treatments. For an explanation of consent in the context of sexual healing, see the previous section about Consent.

Consented agreement on the activities and boundaries used in a session is reached by consulting with the client and discussing sexual healing treatments. This includes a thorough discussion about potential areas where the client might be challenged beyond their ability to receive and process session treatments. During and at the completion of such a discussion on consent, ask questions such as:

"How do you feel about what we've discussed?"

"What are your concerns or questions about what we've discussed?"

"What thoughts or feelings come up for you concerning what we've discussed?"

Desires, Fears, and Boundaries

A way of finding out what someone feels about subjects that are challenging to them is to use the *Desires, Fears, and Boundaries* method.

First, the client is asked, "What is your desire for the session or sexual healing in general?" Their answer will reveal what their intention and goals are for working with the healer. What do they want to accomplish? What symptoms are they seeking relief from?

Next, discuss the client's fears to get an idea of what treatments are appropriate and what level of intensity they are able to work with. Their fears will show you their current limitations and important boundaries that they do not want to cross. These boundaries should always be respected and without attempting to test or adjust them to suit the healer's need to provide a certain type of service or their expectation of what they think the client should be able to tolerate.

Treatments should always be tailored to the client's state of mind and emotional capacity. If a client's fears make it impossible to provide a healer's usual services, then it's either not a good match (and the client should be referred to someone who is more suitable for their needs) or the healer should adjust their service to accommodate where the client is at. A client who is an abuse survivor should never be made to feel they are wrong for having fears about sexual healing or potential harm happening.

When discussing a client's fears it is appropriate for the healer to address each with specific information about how the healer will accommodate them. Either by staying away from certain areas of treatment or by establishing clear procedures and limitations to activities that address the client's fears. If this doesn't allay the client's concerns it would be appropriate to devote time (possibly several sessions) to establish trust and rapport before proceeding further.

After discussing desires and fears, the last phase of the consent discussion is to clearly establish the boundaries that will be in place during healing sessions. This part is last because you want to have the information from their desires and fears first so that the agreed-upon boundaries address these important elements.

Boundaries seek to establish the definitions and limits of activities and interactions that will take place during a healing session. This is where the healer and client agree on a) what will be done, and b) the limits that activity can go, and c) how the activity will be directed—including the client's ability to stop or alter what is happening whenever desired.

Consent is Dynamic

Consent should never be assumed, and it can change with changing circumstances, moods, or emotions. When working with a client, a sexual healer should always ask—rather than assume there is consent. Check in about consent when it appears there has been a shift in the client's attention or presence or an apparent change in their comfort with the activity or treatment.

In initial sessions, spend time with a client to assess and confirm their ability to know and express their truth accurately and freely. The healing alliance mentioned earlier is based on authenticity and trust between the healer and the client. The healer has the responsibility to know (as far as possible) what the client's authentic state of mind and consent is; while the client has the responsibility to know and be aligned (to the best of their ability) with their truth and express it at any time during a session.

Both the client and sexual healer should be prepared for the client's truth about their consent to possibly change at any time before or during a session and immediately accommodate that choice. Session activity should be paused to assess the client's feelings and their ability to clearly know their truth in order to stay current and present with any change to their state of consent.

The sexual healer should try to make sure that a client is not going along with an activity which they are actually averse to due to thinking they are expected to be able to do so or out of trying to be obedient. Therefore, consent needs to be an ongoing conversation and consideration with frequent check-ins and verification of the client's truth with special care in considering whether the client is merely tolerating an activity while not desiring it.

Does this mean that in every situation, activity, and session the client will know what they want and be able to affirmatively express their desire with certainty? No. It can frequently be the case that a client will not be clear about their desire or other feelings. In fact, much of healing involves exploring the unknown. That is what the sexual healer is there for: to be the safe and conscientious steward who is focused on and guided by the client's intention to heal.

A sexual healer shouldn't guess, assume, or follow some formulaic method of treating clients. They should ask the client what they are feeling and what has come up for them. When a client doesn't know what they want—is confused or mentally fragmented—it's a signal to pause and find out what has changed for them and re-determine their consent.

Consent and the Unknown

Are there circumstances when a client will not know what they want but will desire to continue anyway? Yes. However, this should be a conscious decision that acknowledges the uncertainty and incites caution in proceeding with the treatment. As with going on a scary amusement park ride or having an invasive medical treatment, people do difficult or unfamiliar things on purpose to gain a beneficial result that they seek. There can be cases when some aspects of an experience aren't completely desirable, or the client just don't know how they feel about it, yet they are willing to experience it to achieve a greater goal.

- Clients might not know something about themselves or about certain experiences but desire to find out or figure out how they feel about it through experience. Careful exploration and experimentation safely stewarded by the sexual healer can provide the answers the client seeks.
- A client might desire to explore unknown reactions or responses to activities or find out something about their emotional or sensorial capacity which can inform and guide further healing work.
- Sometimes a client desires to know something about themselves and the only way they can do this is to go into an experience to see what their response will be. Use caution and watch the client's reactions and be ready to stop and change the activity to prevent the experience from becoming harmful.

In some cases due to inexperience, a client doesn't know enough to know they desire or don't desire something and must trust beyond their knowledge and be willing to find out. Consent is still required to determine which activity will be used and what will be explored in sessions.

It is sometimes the case that a client may have an expectation that an experience will be harder than it really turns out to be. Or, they may discover they have an appreciation or desire that they didn't know they had until they tried it. In either case, consent is required and the healing facilitator should proceed carefully while observing the client's disposition and reaction to the experience.

When to Check-in to Confirm Consent during a Session

As mentioned previously in the chapter on Consent, there will be organic breaks in a session where the opportunity to check in about the client's emotional state and consent is appropriate. When completing a treatment or exercise and transitioning to the next one is such an opportunity that presents itself in a session.

Additionally, perform a check-in at any point where the session activities or the experience of the client becomes challenging or stretches their comfort area. Sexual Healers will want to anticipate this and look for signs of stress or tension that reveals a pulling back or disconnection. If a client tenses up, holds their breath, clenches, is non-responsive or expresses apprehension, these are signals that the healer should pause and ask about the client's state of being and desire to continue. Whenever these signals manifest, healers should be careful about continuing and make sure that the client is not glossing over their true feelings.

It's important to keep the session at a pace and level of intensity that doesn't overwhelm the client and allows them to assimilate what is being revealed or triggered. To manage this, some sexual healers require their clients to speak a prearranged formulated statement of what they desire or their consent condition.

Having a client make a declarative request for what they want is a good start, but it doesn't completely satisfy the sexual healer's responsibility for accurately understanding their client's consent. If only formulated responses are used it might actually contribute to more confusion and lead to harm. This is because making a formulated statement-request-response may suffice for setting up and commencing treatments or activities but it doesn't account for nondisclosure of discomfort (hiding negative experience or feelings) which can occur after an activity has begun. And, a survivor of sexual trauma may find it hard to speak up, and instead, opt to just keep going—not say anything and suppress their feelings of being out of consent.

If the client is given predetermined and formulated phrases to indicate their consent it can become too easy to just parrot the consent phrase rather than really look deeper for their authentic truth. Instead of using pat phrases or formulated terms for consent, it's better to use open-ended questions and pause for the client's truth to be revealed.

Use open-ended questions or requests like:

- What is coming up for you right now?
- How (or, What) are you feeling?
- What do you need at this moment?
- What questions came up for you? What do you need to be answered?
- Tell me about where you feel challenged in this moment.

Afterward, if the client's consent or desire for an activity or experience hasn't changed then ask whether they are ready to proceed—emphasizing the choice is freely and completely theirs:

- Do you want to take a break or keep going?
- Do you feel complete with this exercise/activity or would you like to explore more?
- Would you like to do something different or does this feel good to you?
- How do you feel about proceeding with _____ (activity)?

If the sexual healer senses there is confusion or conflicted feelings, despite the client's expressed desire to proceed, the healer should state their intuition and suggest a break to give the client space to determine their true feelings and to reconfirm their desire to continue. Only proceed if after confirmation there is no doubt about the client's desire and consent and that their affirmative response reflects their true feelings. Sometimes the healer must use discretion and impose a break or stop a session when they have doubt about a client's true state of desire and consent. A session should be stopped when in spite of the client's affirmative response to continue it is plain to the healer that the experience is too much for the client.

Sexual healers should realize that no matter how they phrase their questions or requests, the client is invariably put in the position of dealing with their personal issues regarding autonomy, safety, and their ability to make choices that reflect their authentic feelings and desire. It is very important for sexual healers to ask open-ended questions and obtain more than perfunctory or routine responses to determine consent during a session.

How often should Consent be affirmed?

Initial sessions should involve establishing trust and rapport to the degree in which a client can access and express their truth to the sexual healer who then responds to it and proceeds only with full and clear consent.

With many clients, it's possible to discover their ability to access and express their truth just by having a conversation that explores their trauma symptoms, and their emotional comfort and its edge. This is a conversation about their symptoms and sexual trauma experiences and the severity of their reaction to situations or experiences (i.e. on a 1 – 10 scale). Find out a) what is happening (their presenting symptoms) and b) how strong a reaction they have to them (their emotional charge). The sexual healer will want to be keenly aware of these edges and give more time and go slower when approaching them to allow the client to take in their experience and feel safe with the process and in expressing their truth about it.

During a sexual healing session, healers should frequently check-in for current consent by asking a client open-ended questions and considering their responses. When the healing alliance has been well established and there are good rapport and trust between client and healer it can be easier to know when a client is tolerating or going along with activities and when there is an authentic "yes" to these.

Attempts to create change too quickly can overwhelm and possibly harm a client. It may take some time to begin to drop their defensive armoring and open to being vulnerable so healing can happen. Care should be taken to proceed with treatments only at a pace that the client can safely integrate their experience.

What's happening Behind the Scenes

At a basic level, being a sexual healer means having the ability to be calm, objective, nonjudgmental, and grounded, while in the presence of another's emotional trauma or activated sexual energy—and to be an adept facilitator of the client's process to release, integrate and heal their wounds. The sexual healer is the steward of the healing session who gently guides the releasing of clenched, contracted emotional, physical, and psychic energy associated with the wounds of emotional and sexual trauma.

The healer's ability to hold a safe and sacred space for the client's process allows the client's emotions and contracted sexual energy to release and integrate. To this end, sexual healers need to understand the existence of—and be able to handle properly—the unexpressed and underlying influences that are present in a sexual healing session.

Sexual healers need to understand as much as is possible their client's state of mind and their emotional load. Basic points to understand include:

- Survivors of sexual abuse or assault are likely to have issues around personal safety and establishing healthy emotional boundaries.
- The fact that the client's trauma is the consequence of a perpetrator disrespecting and overstepping boundaries produces fear and trepidation.
- Clients are likely to have fear and limiting or negative beliefs anywhere they feel vulnerable (e.g. body image and self-esteem) and especially around sex and intimacy.
- Likely, there are more fears and judgments around trusting others, personal space and being touched intimately.
- On top of all of this, clients are generally unfamiliar with sexual healing and what the healing process entails which can add to their confusion and anxiety.

Working with a client exposes the healer to the client's psychological projections (assumptive subjective perceptions or desires held by one person about another without the other person's consent or involvement) associated with their trauma. In addition, the sexual healer's personal process and state of healing and integration of their sexual trauma impacts their ability to provide therapeutic, healthful and harmless service.

Having at least a basic awareness of these influences is important and impacts a client's experience during session treatments. To be a sexual healer is to work with the dark, "shadow" energies of the psyche—both yours and your client's. Sexual energy gets easily encumbered with unconscious, deep wounds because it is vulnerable and powerful at the same time. As a result, this work often evokes strong emotion. Influences that are present in sessions can include enacting roles, fantasies, or expectations which stem from the subconscious of both the client and healer; this phenomenon is known as *transference* and *countertransference.*

Transference and Countertransference

Transference and countertransference are two concepts in psychology which are very important for sexual healers to understand, detect, and be aware of during a session.

The process of working with healing and releasing the trauma of sexual assault/abuse is inherently prone to activate and engage unconscious projections (a person's biased thoughts, feelings or impulses placed onto another person) by both the healer and the client. These projections are understood in psychology as **transference** (the client's experience and assumptions about the healing facilitator) and **countertransference** (the healer's subjective involvement in the therapeutic process). [20]

The client's projections are based on predisposed or biased feelings originating from imprints of significant people (mother, father, other caregivers) or circumstances (abuse trauma) held in the psyche. These projections are placed upon the sexual healer as a role or position the healer fulfills for the client. Ideally, this is the role of a trusted resource for relief, comfort, acceptance, and guidance by a caring, client-focused healer.

Countertransference happens when the sexual healer's projections place the client in a role that attempts to fulfill the healer's illusions. It is important that the sexual healer recognizes when countertransference is present and avoids acting out these projections. Doing so prevents the session from being hijacked in a way that changes its focus from the client's healing process to becoming about the healer's desires or fantasies.

Transference and countertransference in themselves are neither positive nor negative; they are simply facts and ingredients of what the subconscious is processing and are informative to the healer. When transference or countertransference occurs they produce opportunities to understand at a deeper level what is motivating either the client or healer and bring clarity to the healing process.

Michael G. Conner, Psy.D. writes: "Some people refer to transference as a "projection." In this case, you are projecting your own feelings, emotions or motivations onto another person without realizing your reaction is really more about you than it is about the other person. A warm, supportive and kind person could remind you of what you are missing and wanting in your life. You might then idealize that person and begin to see him or her as wonderful beyond belief. Therapists and other health care professionals can also have transference reactions while treating a patient. It's a two-way street. Counter-transference is basically a therapist's "emotional time warp" around their patient's transference. In other words, counter-transference is a therapist's counter-reaction. That's why some therapists think they are falling in love with their patients." [21]

To manage a client's projections, a sexual healer can: reflect, elucidate, or amplify projections back to the client, or choose to contain or absorb them so as to not prematurely interpret them to the client. Sexual healers should monitor their thoughts and desires as well as the client's projections that occur in a session and do their best to not be influenced by these, but use the information to further the client's healing progress. To be able to do this effectively, a healer should be their own first client.

Transference-Countertransference during a session

Training for sexual healers should include how to be aware of transference-countertransference influences during a session.

A transference experience is like a subtext to a conversation which adds an additional meaning, manipulation, or purpose to the primary intent or meaning. The overt communication is the spoken/written content and the covert subtext is found in the way the content is being presented and by the implication of the words which convey an additional meaning—with the intent to manipulate the receiver. A countertransference experience would be the receiver's unconscious reaction to the subtext of the conversation which prompts an imaginative impression that they are, or are becoming, someone who is fulfilling a role, or are representing something important to the other person they are interacting with, such as: savior, teacher, lover, knight, exalted one, etc.—which is an inflation or a fantasy.

In a sexual healing session, this type of transference-countertransference experience could look something like this:

The client feels safe and drops their emotional/psychological armoring to the point which allows them to feel their sensuality and activate their erotic energy. In this state, they also drop their physical armoring which allows their body to begin to move with the sensations of pleasure and energetic pulsing they feel. This will often produce an undulation or stretching, as if to burst invisible straps which have kept the body and erotic energy bound. The client feels their erotic energy and projects their sexual desire onto the healer. The client has successfully tapped into their erotic nature with the facilitation of the sexual healer and is experiencing what it's like to safely activate their sexual energy and wallow in it for a time.

The movements that a client's body makes when its erotic energy is activated and 'running' will look the same as when sharing in a personal sexual experience with an intimate partner. When the sexual healer sees these movements, it unconsciously activates their personal associations with sexual experience. This produces an autonomic response of excitement and adrenaline which carries personal meaning for the healer. If the healer is not aware of what is happening to them there is a danger that the healer will respond personally and cross consent boundaries. During this transference-countertransference influence, the healer is in danger of adopting the role of "lover" and feel that the relationship has shifted from a professional one to a personal one. Whenever a healer realizes they are entertaining a personal fantasy during a session it should be a red flag that they are in danger of succumbing to their projection and the influence of countertransference.

How to tell when countertransference is happening

For sexual healers, having dual awareness is a key ability to utilize during sessions. (See: Deepening and Improving a Sexual Healing Practice) Dual awareness is the ability to hold two concepts, thoughts, ideas, or sets of information, in the mind at the same time. For sexual healers, this ability enables them to remain present and aware of their inner state and any arising influences as well as be aware of their client's emotional state, projections, presence, and ability to integrate their experience.

During sessions, be suspicious of any thoughts that pop into your (the healer's) mind which stray or push the session in a different direction than what was previously discussed and which introduces interactions that push or overrun consent boundaries. Especially when these ideas create fantasy roles or promote personal sexual responses by the healer. These intervening thoughts should be suspect and an alert should go off that something unconscious has been activated and the influence of transference-countertransference is present. Sexual healers should *expect* that such transference-countertransference influences will become active and will present themselves during a session and be alert for these and ready to mitigate their influence.

Transference-countertransference is influential when it is happening while the participants are unconscious to its active presence. Mitigating transference-countertransference influences involves presencing the intervening thought/desire/emotion and consciously considering its validity, its source and its purpose. Thoughts, desires, or emotions that shift the session from professional to personal should trigger immediate action to check what is happening –or about to happen- between the client and healer to make sure professional integrity and the container of informed consent is being maintained. If needed, the healer should pause the session to assess and adjust, or to end the session if they can't recover a professional, objective role and maintain consent integrity.

To deflate or neutralize a client's projection, healers should be able to manage their interaction and alter treatment to preserve right-relationship between client and healer. Sometimes just verbally presencing the projection will pop the bubble—making the unconscious projection be consciously noticed—allowing it to lose its influence on both the client and the healer.

Presencing what is happening for the client offers opportunities to:

a. Become consciously aware of presenting emotions and eros desire—the client's, and for the healer to observe any countertransference impulses.

b. Associated with the above, the sexual healer owns their countertransference impulses, fantasies, and stories with the purpose of deflating these by consciously choosing not to enable them.

c. Assist the client in consciously deepening their connection to eros, their body, and their sexual desire and in creating greater sexual empowerment.

Presencing a client's projections and their sexual desire can take the form of a brief pause and sharing or reporting on 'what's so' or what feels like is not being acknowledged in the moment. The healer's dual awareness should catch countertransference impulses as they arise; and during this break they should do another self-check-in to presence their countertransference realizations—for the purpose of not enabling them.

Countertransference questions to consider:

- What does the client's projection solicit or trigger in the healer? The answer to this will indicate where the healer needs to have more awareness and self-understanding (especially of any unresolved trauma).
- Where in the body is it felt? (genitals 2nd Chakra, head 6th Chakra, heart 4th Chakra) The answer to this question will reveal what part of the psyche and what issues the transference is activating/inflating (genitals = sexual/authority/power; heart = emotional/personal relationships; head = ego/intellectual). Could also activate more than one Chakra.
- What does the thought, desire, emotion or fantasy want to accomplish? Something personal in the healer? Or does it have to do with supporting the client's healing objective?

Things that are for the client will be an aligned "of course" response with no salacious or racy feel to them. Things that emanate from the healer will have an edge to them, a tone of danger, possibly a manic excitement, or a racy "might get caught" thrill feeling.

The above questions provide answers which are useful for self-reflection, understanding, and adjustment in after-session evaluations and reflections. After some experience repeatedly going through these questions after sessions, it will become easier for a healer to recognize when they are happening in real time during a session—and more easily and quickly prevent their influence on the client.

Healer, Heal Thyself

The axiom "healer, heal thyself" especially applies to sexual healers. I have worked with several men and women who sincerely serve as sexual healers and it is noteworthy that they are not immune from needing to process the very same issues regarding intimacy, relationship, and sexuality that their clients face. The fact that sexual healers have dealt with the same issues as their clients is a good thing because that gives them an informed empathy—one based on their own experience.

A sexual healer will likely be triggered by their personal issues while addressing the trauma and issues that their client is working with. Healers should be prepared for this and get the counseling and therapy they need to be consciously aware of, competent with, and as influence-free as possible of their personal issues in sessions with clients.

Before providing sexual healing services to clients, sexual healers should begin with their own issues and trauma wounds. A sexual healer needs to achieve a level of emotional-psychological competency, integration, and wellbeing to prevent their issues from affecting a client's healing process.

It is also important that sexual healers receive feedback and guidance ongoingly—regarding their healing practice experiences, and in processing the emotions that may become activated by clients during sessions. Also, sexual healers should arrange for their own healing sessions and receive energetic and emotional clearing along with somatic treatments to support optimum emotional, energetic, psychological, and physical health.

Cleanly Contributing to Healing

A sexual healing session's ability to provide transformative effects rests largely upon the healer's ability to go into deep empathy (see Informed Empathy) and allow a part of themselves to resonate with where their client is troubled. By so doing, the healer models a tangible new version of the client's condition that reflects the healer's successful, and similar, transformation. [22]

A sexual healer needs to cleanly contribute to a client's healing and integration. Anywhere the healer is blind to their personal psychological or emotional issues will show up in sessions and could limit or divert a client's progress, or could cause harm by adding to the trauma the client is attempting to heal from. [23]

Transference and countertransference, mentioned above, creates an alchemical admixture with results greater than its components. This means that a sexual healer must bring not just their ability to serve in intimate and vulnerable circumstances but also have a trained awareness and intact mental health, which includes competence with handling their personal issues and trauma wounds.

The sexual healer must maintain a balance between identifying with and withdrawing from the client's projections. Their ability to remain neutral when provoked to identify with a projection can be an important step in a client's healing process by allowing them to see the projection and work to release it.

Feedback and Mentorship

Additional training, and ongoing self-reflection and evaluation, as well as working with a more experienced mentor will aid a sexual healer in responding to a client's transference effectively.

To manage a client's transference and their own countertransference, healers must:

- Become adept with having dual awareness that monitors their inner experience along with a client's projections.
- Consciously respond to transference-countertransference to steward sessions in a useful direction so transformation and healing can be reached.

To help sexual healers competently handle transference-countertransference issues it's very important that they receive as part of their training—and ongoingly—feedback and mentorship by an experienced sexual healer, or a qualified therapist or counselor. It is also a good practice to have post-session reviews, and make note of the projections which were perceived and their influence on the healer and client.

Informed Empathy and Acceptance

A key concept for sexual healers is the implementation of informed empathy—which is the ability to understand another person from their point of view, informed by the healer's similar experiences. Another key is the healer's ability to accept and meet a client where they are at emotionally and psychologically without assuming or imposing expectations of where they should be.

On a significant level, whatever a healer doesn't have integrated or understood concerning their own psychological and emotional baggage is unconsciously brought into sessions with clients. If a sexual healer isn't working on their issues and becoming increasingly aware of their influence then they are likely contaminating the client's process with their personal issues. A sexual healer isn't required to be perfect, however they should be adept with conscientiously managing their personal complexes or issues and any sexual trauma wounds and be able to keep those from negatively impacting a client.

Adequate and Appropriate Training

Competence comes from the right application of training and experience that supports the healing alliance. Sexual Healers should begin by getting all the training they possibly can from private sessions, workshops, lectures, books and responsible internet resources. Follow that up with some type of an internship or apprenticeship working with a mentor in several sessions to gain initial experience. Choose a mentor who has a good amount of experience and regularly consult with them.

How much training is adequate? Certainly, it would seem that attending one workshop on yoni healing would not by itself qualify someone to be a sexual healer. A series of private tutoring and/or group classes with guided training sessions that are reviewed by qualified instructors similar to other alternative healing certification programs is appropriate.

Ideally, new sexual healers would have supervised co-facilitated sessions as part of their training. In some cases, sexual healers may have previous experience from training in other healing modalities which can enhance their qualifications.

Specific areas of training for sexual healing should include the following:

- The body's subtle energy system and its function (Nadis, Chakras, subtle bodies)
- The physical body including the sympathetic and parasympathetic nervous system, muscles, skeleton, skin, trigger or pressure points, and erogenous locations
- STD-STI exposures
- Sexual response cycle
- Breath-work and how it affects energy, physiology, and state of mind
- Basic understanding of the psyche

   a. The healer's personal issues and trauma wounds
   b. Transference-countertransference
   c. Effects of trauma and how the mind processes traumatic experiences

- Psychological or emotional shock, fragmentation, acute stress reaction, and dissociative states.
- Ethical Best Practices that protect the client's right to mental, emotional, psychological, and physical safety and confidentiality.

Tantra Sexual Healer Training

There are some Tantra based Sexual Healing Schools which offer training courses, workshops, or retreats. Be careful when attending and participating in these types of events; there have been several sexual assault and rape allegations made against some of the most prominent Tantra schools and their leaders/teachers/healers.

Any Tantra training that addresses sexual healing for clients should include significant coverage of Consent and provide training in sexual healing session ethics that maintains consent integrity and protects the client from attitudes and behavior that causes sexual assault.

Training for Tantric/Sexual Healers should also include understanding transference-countertransference and how shadow elements become active and how to mitigate their influence, as well as training in introspective self-reflection and self-awareness/reporting—including getting feedback from a mentor or coach.

STD-STI Exposures

Many sexual healing treatments or activities don't require genital touching or invasive techniques or removing clothing covering the genital area. When no invasive treatments or genital touching is included in session treatments, exposure to STD/STI is no more likely than when getting a massage or being examined by a clinician or doctor. If session activities are limited to those that avoid contact with bodily fluids or possibly infected areas of the skin then there is no need for the disclosure of personal sexual health by the client or healer.

However, there are sexual healing activities where exposure to an STD/STI is possible. In these cases, the sexual healer and the client need to have a frank conversation disclosing any STD/STI health conditions.

In harmony with safer sex practices designed to prevent STD/STI exposure and transmission, sexual healers should use a barrier that prevents contact with any infected areas. Any activities that could come in contact with infected areas or bodily fluids should be covered and protected from direct contact.

When invasive treatments are used (vaginal or anal), a sexual healer will usually wear medical examination gloves (these should *always* be worn whenever the healer has hangnails, cuts or sores). When there is no exposure to STD/STI transmission gloves might not be worn—especially when the treatment requires greater touch sensitivity. However, the decision to not wear gloves must include the client's consent.

HPV

The most common sexually transmitted infection, by some estimates present in up to 80% of sexually active people, is HPV. [24] HPV is a virus that is spread through intimate skin-to-skin contact and can be passed during vaginal, anal and oral sex.

HPV can cause genital warts and in some cases cause certain types of cervical cancer. HPV is transmitted via infected skin, on and around the genitals. Using a condom greatly reduces exposure, however, HPV can infect areas not covered by a condom. Most types of HPV are harmless and do not have noticeable symptoms, which is why most people don't know that they carry HPV or what type they have. There is no test for men to know if they carry it.

For sexual healers, genital to genital touching is not normally part of session activities and 99% of treatments do not involve mutual genital connection. However, in some sexual healing sessions (especially Tantric Healing, or at Tantric "puja" events) sitting together in Yab-Yum position (lap sitting with legs wrapped around each other) is utilized as a breathing and energy balancing exercise. Doing so brings the client's and healer's genitals into close proximity of each other. If both the client's and healer's genitals are uncovered when in Yab-Yum position there can be an exposure to HPV transmission.

Motivations to Serve

Why do you want to be a sexual healer?

It's very important to be clear regarding the motivations and reasons for serving in this extremely sensitive, vulnerable, and potent field that is deeply intimate, healing, and transformative. Many sexual healers desire to provide comfort and relief to others because they wish to share what they have experienced in their path of healing and a return to wholeness, sexual, and sensual empowerment.

If someone is recovering from sexual abuse or trauma and desires to serve others as a sexual healer, they owe it to themselves and their clients to get a qualified and objective opinion on whether they have made enough progress with their personal healing to truly be of aid and service to others.

Facilitating sexual healing is not simply about being able to *be sensual* in the presence of a stranger—a client. One's ability to be sensual with a client is only one of many elements used to address the intimate issues that impact a client's wounded or blocked sexuality. To show up able to engage another's erotic energy is only opening the door to addressing a client's sexual healing needs.

A person's motivation to serve as a sexual healer is often influenced by the deep desires of their subconscious. A sexual healer needs to be very clear about, and familiar with, their emotional wounds and 'personal shadow' (as best as they are able to). If they are not, they risk being affected by these and affecting their client's experience negatively as issues emerge to which they unconsciously react.

In the Sacred Sexuality and neo-Tantra worlds, one resource for motivation to serve as a sexual healer comes from the popular perception of the roles that ancient priestesses (and priests) performed in sacred ceremonies—that apparently included sexual acts. [25] The obvious warning here is to watch out for romanticizing and inflating what is known with what is conjecture at the risk of performing an idealized character —making the session about the performance instead of the client's healing.

The Temple Priestess Role Model

Sumerian, Babylonian, and other ancient cultures throughout the Mediterranean, Middle East, and North Africa had a provocative feature included in their worship of the Great Goddess which many sexual healers take inspiration from today. These women, who were known by titles such as Hierodule, Qadishtu, and Harimtu, lived and served in the temple centers of Isis, Ishtar, Inanna, and Aphrodite— where religious ceremony and sexual energy were utilized together without social prejudice or conflict. [26]

An example of such a priestess is found in the Gilgamesh[27] story, the oldest written epic known to humanity. In it, a Hierodule (sexual priestess) plays a key role in awakening the unevolved, unawakened masculine in the uncivilized Gilgamesh to a higher consciousness, psychological maturation and integration. [28]

In contrast with today, these ancient cultures viewed sexual intercourse as a sacred way of empowering ritual and ceremony. To the ancients, the temple priestess and male patron taking part in these sacred ceremonies experienced something akin to the Catholic belief of transubstantiation,[29] —the ceremonial, miraculous transformation of sacramental wine into the blood of the Christ and biscuit wafers transformed to become his body.

In these ceremonies, the priestess and her lover would become representatives of the divine couple who copulate for the purpose of communing with the divine and thereby acquire their gifts of healing, wisdom, insight, blessings and abundance, protection, and salvation. Sexual ecstasy and pleasure were the sacraments of their sacred communion.

In modern times, sexual healers can use the inspiration of the Qadishtu-priestess to serve as the impetus for divine inspiration, transformation, and higher eros. Modern Qadishtu have the ability to awaken men and women to higher states of consciousness and transcendent sexual experiences in addition to helping them to heal from sexual abuse and trauma. The obvious difference in applying the Qadishtu example in modern times is that sexual intercourse is rarely, if ever applied with clients. However, the utilization and application of sexual energy and sensual pleasure for the purposes of healing is similar.

Some women can get caught up in a 'participation mystique' or a fantasy about being a priestess or a goddess who is to be served— having power over others by virtue of a title or their sexual openness. For some women, the fantasy of being a sacred prostitute and fulfilling the role of an ancient priestess can be a projection of unresolved personal issues which are likely to adversely affect clients. Men have their version of participation mystique also, falling into fantasies of being a great lover capable of satisfying many women, or as a savior-healer-knight in shining armor rescuing a damsel in distress by satisfying her sexually, etc.

To get clear about one's motivation and desire to be a sexual healer, seek the help of an experienced personal coach, counselor or therapist—not just peers who might not have enough objectivity. Someone with an authentic calling won't over-romanticize or over-identify with the role or title of Priestess but will focus on serving the spiritual, emotional, and sexual wellbeing of their clients. Finding a balance that includes a conscious embodiment of the ancient Qadishtu–priestesses model and an adept understanding of the human psyche and trauma wounding will enable modern priestess-sexual healers to be a genuine benefit to their clients.

Of course, it's not necessary to relate to the ancient priestess-healer archetype to be an adept sexual healer. It is equally valid to have a modern, and secular interest in aiding people to heal, understand, and experience their sexuality at a more integrated level. In both instances, a prospective sexual healer needs to examine their motives and any illusions they might be unaware of affecting their ability to effectively and harmlessly serve their clients.

Get Your Ego Out of the Way

The Ego is the conscious self, [30] and in its immature, inflated, or unconscious state is self-focused and concerned with making itself appear to be more, or other than, what it actually is. When someone is being influenced by their inflated ego they have a distorted perception that is concerned with preserving appearances and in playing a role or a projection of oneself.

When the Ego is unmoderated by one's higher, spiritual nature, a person's focus is more superficial and lacks a depth of presence. When spiritual awareness leads the Ego there is a right-relationship with it that places a healer more completely in the present moment focusing on serving the client's needs over their own.

Egoic Performance and Self-Judgment

One way that an unbalanced Ego can effect healing sessions is in setting up accomplishment and performance expectations. It's important that the healer let go of expectations for the client's experience. If a sexual healer is preoccupied with "am I doing this right?" from an egoic performance perspective, then this critical self-judgment will infect the healer's presence and treatments. Taking satisfaction in helping to facilitate healing is fine, it is important to maintain a high standard of competency, just don't let it become a pursuit of giving star performances that are about stroking the Ego.

Spirit's Role

Being attuned to a spiritual awareness and perspective will aid sexual healers to remain harmless in their service. Spiritual beliefs that are focused on helping people heal and that inspire personal transformation and growth create a personal moral compass which guides a healer's thoughts, desires, and behavior.

A sexual healer will have a repository of experience, intuition, and knowledge, developed through personal experience, education and training, meditation and spiritual practice. The sexual healer draws from this accumulated resource with spirit's guidance during a session.

Spirit's guidance will be focused on the client's healing and wellbeing and won't be overly concerned about 'performance' or trying to fulfill the healer's personal interests or fantasies. When healers are committed to understanding their personal emotional baggage and projections; and have processed and integrated these, it is much easier to discern what guidance is coming from spirit and what is coming from their Ego.

In addition, it's essential that the healer honors the client's spiritual condition and unique connection to spirit's guidance for them—a client's intuition can provide key insight into facilitating healing and should be welcomed.

The sexual healer's unconscious shadow creates great potential for harm to occur if there is no opportunity or outlet for discovering, processing and understanding it. Spiritual practice and a spiritual mindset will encourage understanding and processing of emotional trauma. With spirit's help in revealing and understanding previously hidden influences, these are integrated into conscious awareness, and are then disarmed of their impulsive power.

The sexual healer's spiritual connection is the conduit by which the healing container and the healing alliance with the client are kept clear of personal shadow aspects that can negatively affect the client. In addition to training, personal work and mentoring, it is important for a sexual healer to maintain a spiritual practice of meditation and introspection so they can readily and clearly see their ego's influence and know how their wounds and shadow aspects are affecting them.

The essence of serving as a sexual healer is non-personal—having a transpersonal and spiritual foundation focused on benefiting others. Adept sexual healers develop the ability to go beyond their ego's need to dominate or be the authority and instead align their awareness to what spirit is directing them to do in concert with the client's spiritual guidance. Trust that the client has sought you out because Spirit has guided them to work with you due to your unique combination of experience and awareness.

Interacting with Clients

"Running Sexual Energy" with a Client

Running sexual energy means to ignite sexual energy and encourage it to maintain a charge while circulating or flowing throughout the client's body-mind perception. It is a procedure that helps a sexual healer see where a client's sexual energy might be stuck or contracted and not flowing freely. Sexual energy that flows freely increases mind-body awareness and integration and enhances the client's sense of sensual embodiment, and their ability to experience and express sensually.

Running sexual energy will typically involve igniting sexual energy through erotic touch, breath work, and movement to encourage the energy to flow. This typically means that sexual energy is experienced beyond the genital area, extending up the spine to the heart, head, and down arms and legs; and in this way, the energy can be conceived as flowing in a circuit.

In most cases, igniting sexual energy can be done through breath-work and body movement alone. Some practitioners include touching a client's body sensually, (in some cases their genitals) as part of assisting the client in activating their sexual energy. Some sexual healers may also allow mutual touch while running sexual energy to encourage the client's experience and ability to sense and participate in the energetic flow. If mutual touch is allowed, it will normally be limited to non-sexual touch of the healer by the client. It is vital for sexual healers and clients to discuss the subject of intimate touch, its limits and whether it is one-way or mutual as part of setting the intention and container for healing sessions. (See also: Erotic Enrichment sessions)

Intimate Touch

Full body sensual massage is a frequent treatment used in sexual healing to relax the body and activate erotic energy. Anytime hands-on healing treatments are included they increase the possibility for a client to feel emotionally confused and can trigger their trauma wounds. With sexual healing, the fact that this touch can often be to erogenous areas and is activating sexual energy creates an additional need for conscientious care to keep from unintentionally harming a client.

Touching a client can also create confusion if the client, or practitioner, or both become emotionally enmeshed and identify with their projections regarding the other. In the book Touching: Body Therapy and Depth Psychology, Deldon Anne McNeely Ph.D. speaks to analysts about patient transference and the therapist-client power dynamic: [31]

"In touching a patient we very easily open up the possibility of preverbal transferences. That is, by physical contact when the patient is in a regressed, non-defended state, we set up conditions whereby the patient may fuse with the analyst as an infant would, at such an early level that it cannot be conceptualized in words. Intense dependency needs are often evoked which are not entirely in the patient's awareness and are not spoken of unless the therapist can bring them forth. Sometimes these early needs can appear to the patient as a strong sexual attraction to the therapist. Skill and experience on the part of the therapist are needed to discern the patient's true needs.

The misuse of power, especially with regard to sexual acting out, reveals the shadow of analysis."

While McNeely is addressing psychiatric analysts/therapists, her explanation of pre-verbal transference exposures and the triggering of fantasy delusions that these can activate is relevant for sexual healers to consider, especially since sexual healers work with sexual energy. (See also: Transference-Countertransference)

When the sexual healer has a practice of self-examination and reviews sessions with a mentor it is less likely that significant problems will arise. Cultivating this self-knowledge can be a long process and no amount of reading by itself can take the place of working with an experienced counselor or mentor.

Nudity in a Session

Nudity in a session, by either the client or sexual healer, takes a healing session to another level of intimacy and creates a profound impact on session activities and the atmosphere of the session container.

When both the healer and client are nude together in a session, it activates an unconscious impression that the session's interactions are more personal. Nudity, on its own sets off a cascade of unconscious physiological and psychological reactions which activate personal sex response patterns—effecting objectivity and mental clarity.

Nudity in a session makes a statement and characterizes the session as something closer to being a "date" or a more relaxed and personal interaction, which can create more exposure for consent boundaries being confused or crossed. Before including nudity in a session, the healer and client will want to discuss the additional influence and impact that will be produced and understand for what purpose nudity is included.

Being nude in a session can be very challenging for a survivor of sexual abuse. When a sexual healer is nude it can confuse the client, calling them to participate with more personal interaction—or to allow the healer to be more personal with them. Any of these conditions could trigger a survivor and cause emotional harm.

Why would nudity be included in a session?

There should never be an expectation that a client be nude for sexual healing sessions—or comply in order to receive certain treatments. If a client doesn't want to be unclothed for a treatment that the healer normally applies to nude clients then the treatment should be altered or another treatment substituted in its place. The client's desire for and state of readiness and ability to receive appropriate treatments while nude should be carefully considered and discussed before including nudity in a session. Nudity is certainly not appropriately routine for sexual healing sessions and should be a point of discussion during consent conversations about session activity boundaries.

There are breathing and movement exercises which can be used in sexual healing sessions and which don't require the client to be unclothed. And these should be used with clients initially, especially with sexual abuse survivors. When adding hands-on healing and sensual touch to a session, it can be beneficial for the client to disrobe to allow better access to the body—and yet may remain covered by draping (e.g. massage draping) if desired.

When a client has worked with a healer for several sessions and there is rapport and trust established between them—and as part of the client's healing process in feeling more empowered and safe—the client might feel inclined to be fully nude. This will often be the case while receiving a sensual massage. Without draping, a client's nude body exposed to the air can heighten the sensual experience.

In sexual healing sessions, and especially with new clients, it isn't necessary or appropriate for the healer to be nude. If the healer is nude, it will send the wrong message and intention to the client and characterize the session as a personal sexual interaction—causing confusion and possible harm to the client. Sexual healing treatments don't require the healer to be nude to facilitate them. Sexual healers (or Tantric Healers) are nurturing egoic fantasies if they think their nudity is essential to include in a session with a client.

Mutual Sexual Gratification

For sexual healing sessions, one-way touch with the healer touching and the client receiving the touch fits with accepted treatment practice in traditional and most alternative healing modalities. This kind of contact and boundaries supports the client's pace, capacity, and ability to integrate their experience. Mutual sexual pleasuring is typically associated with intimate personal relationships and could be confusing to the client and possibly be harmful if included in a sexual healing session.

It is important to remember why the client has chosen to have a sexual healing session—they desire to receive a transformative healing experience. In no way should a healing session be considered "a date," a purchase of sex, or a way to meet the healer's sex fantasy, relationship, or intimacy needs. If a sexual healer feels that their clients are coming to them to fulfill the healer's personal sexual desires, then there is a fundamental misunderstanding by the sexual healer of the healing alliance.

While sexual healers experience great satisfaction in facilitating growth and healing, and they might also benefit from revelations and truths presented during a session, these are secondary to the prime intention of serving the client's healing transformation, wellbeing, and highest good—and not their personal sexual needs.

Case Study: Ejaculating on a Client

In 2011, a thread in an email group discussing sexual healing topics revealed that a male sexual healer was ejaculating on his client as part of a shamanic sex magic ritual utilized in his sexual healing practice—without prior disclosure or consent by his client.

The specific details of the scenarios or the efficacy of this practice notwithstanding, the bigger question concerns exposing a client to the possible harm caused by enacting such a provocative procedure which is unannounced and unprepared for. Without prior informed consent, these reported actions are most likely experienced as assaultive, and not healing or transformative.

In a sexual healing session, it's not necessary or advisable for a male healer to ejaculate. In my many years of being a sexual healer, I have never seen the need or appropriateness of ejaculating during a sexual healing session. In my opinion, if a daka ejaculates during a sexual healing session, it means he has lost an essential level of objectivity and his sexual arousal has overtaken him and he has been caught up in some fantasy of mutual sexual pleasuring.

Allowing for special circumstances where an unusual or obscure sexual healing method is being used that includes ejaculation of semen onto the client as part of a ritual or ceremony, the daka should at the very least—and prior to the session—have a thorough discussion of the subject and the intended action and affirm consent before initiating such a procedure.

Male sexual healers have the incredible opportunity to show up in their elevated, sacred masculine nature that steadfastly supports the client's healing intention and the right to safety and wellbeing. By so doing, a woman can feel safe enough to let go, release, and heal. After that, she can feel enough safety and trust to begin to strengthen her erotic prowess until she regains her sexual autonomy and confidence. Unexpected and unsanctioned surprises—such as ejaculation—shatter the trust that a woman feels and subverts the intention of healing that she desires.

Likewise, female sexual healers are privileged to represent the feminine force in facilitating healing with their clients. Men under the care of a female healer must be able to trust her enough to open their protected emotions—letting go of their pain, shame and regret. If they feel their trust is misplaced or betrayed by a female healer playing a role who is not present with the client's condition and needs, they will contract and retreat into their protective shell—adding another story to their narrative about being betrayed by the feminine.

Tantra Lessons and Tantric Healing Sessions

Some sexual healers are also trained in Tantra and incorporate Tantric energy techniques in their sessions. Tantra is a very powerful spiritual-sexual-science which understands and works with sexual energy with profound effects. Tantra is also associated with a community of people who share in Tantra events with group activities often called a *puja* (Sanskrit: prayer, ritual, an act of worship) which creates a more personal, and social type of atmosphere. Typically, in these experiences, there is liberal sensuality and greater sexual openness.

In these settings, and with the Tantra communal feel, sexual healing or Tantra lesson sessions can create confusion regarding boundaries. Things that may happen at Tantra workshops, parties, or pujas in a personal environment are not necessarily appropriate in a sexual healing session or Tantra lesson.

Is it ever acceptable to have consensual sex with a Tantra client/ student?

When the Tantra teacher/healer and the client/subject are not already in a personal relationship the answer is: NO, sex is not appropriate. Consenting adults who decide they agree to have intercourse can, of course, do whatever they want to together, as long as there is mutual consent. But when there is a professional teacher or healer relationship, and without prior informed consent, it is inappropriate for the teacher/healer to have sex with a client.

Tantra lessons or healing sessions between a teacher/healer and client/subject are not a "date" opportunity and not the appropriate setting for the teacher/healer to get their personal sexual needs met. Any Tantra teacher/healer who thinks that having sex with clients is an expected part of a session is deluding themselves and causing harm to their client.

There are some Tantra teachers who will provide a Tantric "initiation" ceremony that can include sexual intercourse with a client. However, this is and should be a rare occurrence and only after thorough disclosure and discussion—and only with wholehearted informed consent. AND, this is definitely not the case when a Tantric teacher or healer shifts the focus of a session and decides it's time for him to get his pleasure and assaults/rapes his client/student (as has been alleged in some cases).

It should never be the case where a teacher/healer has sex with a client impromptu during a session—even with the client's consent— because the client is likely in a diminished capacity to responsibly make that choice due to being under the influence of Tantric thrall or somatic trance from the session.

One critical ability a Tantra teacher/healer must have is to maintain the container of consent even if the sexual energy in the session becomes extremely potent. Tantra teachers/healers cannot succumb to personal desires and cross this line and expect there won't be harm created.

Sexual Intercourse in Sexual Healing Treatments

Sexual healing regularly occurs without intercourse as a session feature or treatment and the overwhelming majority of sexual healing treatments do not include intercourse with a client. Intercourse is not necessary and in most cases is not appropriate and should rarely –if at all– be considered as a treatment.

Sexual intercourse has tremendous significance—bearing emotional, physical, and psychological effects for both participants. Intercourse can potentially impact a woman's psyche more profoundly because she is the one being penetrated and because she has likely been a sexual assault survivor. To include sexual intercourse in a sexual healing session marks an important development of profound significance and should only be included after thorough clearheaded consideration and consent.

In a professional and responsible practice of sexual healing, intercourse with a client would not be routinely or indiscriminately included in a session. Certainly, intercourse would not be spontaneously offered or promoted during a session—and never as a "reward" or expectation by the sexual healer.

Some women who have worked with sexual healers have shared with me that they consider experiencing sexual intercourse in their sessions with a *daka* (male sexual healer) essential to their healing process. They report that without it, they wouldn't have reached the level of healing they needed. Additionally, couples in a personal intimate relationship who are trained in sexual healing and include intercourse in their sessions with each other can also experience deep levels of healing. I take from this that under the right conditions there is no doubt regarding the potentially positive impact of including intercourse in a sexual healing session and healing program. However, intercourse with a client should never be routinely used as a treatment and should only be considered in specific and rare cases.

Ultimately it is a personal decision between the sexual healer and the client to be consciously made together. If it is carefully considered and weighed against potential emotional or psychological harm—and then still considered to be an essential aspect of the client's growth or healing—then who is to say it is not appropriate for that client?

Enmeshment, Codependency, and Pseudo Relationships

Due to the emotional-psychological-physical intimacy, vulnerability, and openness present in sexual healing sessions, a sexual healer faces added exposure to becoming emotionally enmeshed or attached to their client(s) and vice versa.

The ideal relationship with a client is one of transpersonal care, empathy, emotional–psychological support, and endearing familiarity without infatuation or connecting in a way that diminishes the healer's ability to be sufficiently neutral and objective to facilitate positive transformation for the client.

A sexual healer pursuing personal needs for intimacy, relationship or sexual fulfillment during sexual healing sessions does a disservice to the client and runs a great risk of becoming enmeshed in an emotionally confusing and distorted relationship. The point in which a healer's personal sexual patterns take over can go unrecognized and infect and detour the session—bringing confusion or harm to the client. Sexual healers must be able to maintain the ability to consciously self-monitor and moderate their feelings and behavior to avoid pursuing personal relationship needs or acting on their sexual desires.

Having a mentor and getting regular feedback, along with maintaining dual awareness, self-observation, and introspection, will help a sexual healer remain effective and provide optimum service to their client. A regular practice of inquiring within and seeking mental-emotional clarity will help make sure interactions with a client are not confused with personal agendas.

A sexual healer must be able to monitor their emotional state and check within to see what if any, unconscious patterns, schemes, or ulterior motives may be active. These must be cleared and the ability to remain emotionally neutral and objective nurtured—while being present, engaged and available to the client.

In addition to the above, as a professional, it is unethical to create pseudo-personal relationships for commercial gain. When a sexual healer creates a false impression of a deeper connection than what is actually their truth it sets up an energetic conflict which is likely to spill out into overt confusion and harm when the client realizes the appearance of a personal relationship has been used as merely an income resource.

The large gray area here is with informal or friendship relationships and sexual healing sessions. Just because there is no monetary exchange for a sexual healing session doesn't lessen the need to be clear and responsible with one's intentions, feelings, and behavior.

To the contrary, when occurring informally, or between friends, there can be an even greater possibility of misunderstanding and confusion of feelings, and all the more reason to be clear about the feelings between the client and healer and the intention for the sexual healing session.

Energetic Care for Yourself and Your Client

Sexual healers work in the realm of life force energy—also known as chi, prana, and kundalini—which animates and supports the physical body. Studies of subtle energy agree with ancient Yogic knowledge of energy fields that radiate beyond the physical limitations of the body which can interact with energy fields belonging to other people (i.e., clients). This interaction can be harmonious and congenial or it can also leave discordant residue and disruptive imprints that can affect the vitality and clarity of a sexual healer's energy field. [32]

Clients are carrying and processing emotional and psychological wounds affecting the most intimate and vulnerable aspects of who they know themselves to be. They struggle with issues of self-esteem, trust, intimacy, autonomy, and sexuality, and they can be predisposed to enmeshment and projections that can have a negative energetic impact on the healer they are working with. Establishing a protection protocol or ritual for energetic, spiritual and psychological clarity will help to clear away any energetic residue from clients and prepare the session room for another client.

Sexual healers can be affected by their client's energy due to the intimate and empathetic engagement during a session. These energetic entanglements or attachments can eventually accumulate to the point of causing one to feel sick or depressed. To manage this and protect themselves, sexual healers should perform an energy clearing and shielding ritual before and after each session with a client.

Any effective ritual or ceremony (i.e. chants or mantras) which establishes and maintains a strong protective awareness sphere that keeps the healer's energy field clear and unencumbered during and after a healing session should be practiced. As part of their training, sexual healers need to learn as much as they can about subtle energy, clearing and charging energy fields and energy centers (aka "Chakras") as well as grounding and releasing energy that is not aligned or compatible with the healer's energy field.

Energetic interaction and boundaries

Sexual healers should also be conscious of how their energy is projected into their environment and especially how it effects their clients—as well as how a client's energy can impact the sexual healer. Healers do well to realize which of their Chakras is active and where their energy is emanating from and where it is interacting with the client's energy. Sexual energy covertly directed by the sexual healer to a client can be received as an intrusion or assault. Sexual healers should monitor their energy and make sure they are not energetically assaulting their clients.

Sexual abuse survivors frequently have an impacted energy field resulting from their struggle with the emotional and psychological wounds they carry. Very often they also have no idea of how their impacted energy projects and affects other people. It's not necessary that clients be informed about this, but it is important that the sexual healer is aware and has methods to transmute and release the impact of their client's energy when it occurs.

It's a good practice to regularly clear energetic debris from your energy field throughout the day, and especially between sessions with clients. Perform an energy clearing and balancing ritual using sage, crystals, or some other method you know which clears any energetic projections that have impacted you. Pay special attention to your hands and the Chakras located on the palms if you touch your client using your hands or fingers.

Role-Playing Sexual Fantasies

Role Play, an aspect of Gestalt Therapy,[33] is an accepted therapeutic counseling method[34] that often brings unique insights. Role play in sessions can be useful and effective depending on the client's condition. There are therapists and sexual healers who do good work with carefully and responsibly implementing role play. However, because role play activates unconscious psychological responses, additional care should be taken—and role play should not be indiscriminately used with unprepared clients.

Exploring the fulfillment of sexual fantasies can certainly be part of sexual healing. However, some sexual healers advertise exotic fantasy roles to grab the attention of potential clients in a commercially competitive environment. In other cases, if a sexual healer uses role play with clients for personal fantasy fulfillment there can be a counterproductive effect which reinforces delusions or fantasies. By assuming the role of a sex goddess, priestess, or sexual muse, essentially becoming a *sex-fairy* granting wishes, a sexual healer risks bypassing real transformation and healing. Role play misapplied or misused as a seduction tool or as marketing hype misses the point of sexual healing.

Business Ethics in Sexual Healing

Money'$ Influence

Fees for sexual healing sessions can range from small amounts to several hundred dollars depending on the session length and the healer's experience and qualifications. At the moment, there seems to be a range from $200+ an hour for female sexual healers and $100 an hour for male sexual healers.

Women in particular who serve as sexual healers are in high demand for their services by men who are willing to pay extravagant amounts for the experience of being with them. This can create a moral challenge and distraction for some women due to the lucrative aspect of men seeking exotic sex experiences and not necessarily sexual healing. It's a consideration that each sexual healer has to contemplate and clarify regarding what their sacred service will, or will not be about and what motivates their service.

I have heard some dakinis express in gleeful, greedy amazement, how much they can charge men who are willing to pay for what amounts to a sex fantasy experience. Whatever levels of "healing" or enrichment these men may experience—it seems counterproductive to foster the dynamic of exploitation. For any sexual healer to leverage their sexuality for the purpose of monetarily exploiting their clients' desires is misguided.

Sexual healing practitioners who consciously and purposefully facilitate sexual healing for their clients are primarily focused on their client's reason for having the session—healing, and not on how much money they are making. Money is an important part of the energy exchange between the client and healer. However, let money be a secondary consideration to the primary purpose of transpersonal service to aid others to heal and return to an empowered state of wellbeing. A sexual healer should charge reasonable rates that promote equitable client-healer relationships.

Marketing and Getting Clients

The axiom "You get who you market for" certainly holds true in the field of sexual healing. The type of clients that respond and the expectations that they have are heavily influenced by the invitation they see—the way in which sexual healing services are presented and what is being offered. This is the first link in the chain of events leading to sexual healing where integrity and ethical behavior impact the client's experience and could cause confusion or harm if not presented truthfully and transparently.

In some cases, advertising for clients, workshops, seminars, classes, or lessons in sexuality, sexual healing, sexual enrichment, or guidance about sexual energy, there has been an appeal to the salaciousness of sex by using revealing or alluring pictures or gratuitously salacious statements. Often in these cases, the appeal is mostly to men who are seeking to fulfill a sex fantasy or ego gratification through sex. Some of these advertisements list sexual healing as one of the benefits, or purposes of the session, proclaiming the healing benefits of orgasm. This hyped up sexuality is meant to grab attention and ensnare client's desires.

There is certainly a place for the pure enjoyment of sex for sex sake—and for some men there can be a sense of relief or healing to experience sexual fantasy fulfillment. However, it would be counterproductive and possibly traumatic for a client to enter into what they thought was a healing session and be faced with having sex, or hyped up sexual interactions. If a sexual healer is thinking: "What clients really want, but are afraid to ask for, is sex and so they will be grateful for getting it" it is the healer's delusional fantasy and it does not serve the best interest of their client. Acting on this thinking is likely to re-wound and traumatize the client.

Sexual Healers might also provide erotic enrichment sessions— which focus more on sensual rehabilitation, revitalization, and gaining experience and empowerment. It's important for sexual healers who provide erotic enrichment to determine what it is the client is looking for in the requested session. It's certainly possible that enrichment can happen in a healing session and healing can happen in an enrichment session. However, the focus and trajectory of the session should not be other than what the client is there to receive and has consented to.

Marketing and advertising for your services will also expose you to scrutiny by law enforcement in areas where sexual healing is considered illegal prostitution or pandering. How you present yourself and the "invitation" you use will go a long way towards getting either the right attention that brings you clients who are a good fit or the wrong attention that puts you in a law enforcement spotlight and possible arrest. So consider your marketing strategy and your invitation carefully. Focusing on "education" and "alternative healing" with as much consideration for the legal requirements for healing businesses in your local area may help you avoid unwanted attention and prosecution.

Legal Exposures

Sexual Healers face possible arrest on criminal charges (criminal liability) or as a defendant in civil lawsuits (legal liability) and should be aware of these exposures and what they mean.

Criminal Liability

Criminal liability is the legal exposure to being arrested for breaking the law. With sexual healing, most often the laws used to prosecute healers are about *pandering* and *prostitution*.

- **Pandering** is defined as the catering to or exploitation of the weaknesses of others, especially to provide gratification for others' desires. Pandering penalizes various acts by intermediaries who engage in the commercial exploitation of prostitution and are aimed at those who, as agents, promote prostitution rather than against the prostitutes themselves. [35]
- **Prostitution** generally means the commission by a person of any natural or unnatural sexual act, deviate sexual intercourse, or sexual contact for monetary consideration or another thing of value. [36]

Legal Liability

Legal Liability is your exposure to being sued for causing harm to someone.

- **Legal Liability** means legal responsibility for one's acts or omissions. Failure of a person or entity to meet that responsibility leaves him/her/it open to a lawsuit for any resulting damages or a court order to perform (as in a breach of contract or violation of statute). [37]

You could think of legal liability as being responsible for someone slipping and falling while on your premises because you failed to clean up a spill on the floor. For sexual healers, it may also involve mental/emotional anguish or claims of physical harm due to activities or procedures used during a session.

Protections against Legal Liability consist of "Hold Harmless" agreements (for contracts) and liability insurance which has different forms:

1. Premises liability, protects the property owner from claims that a person was injured on the premises (i.e. "slip and fall" exposures).
2. Professional liability protects against "errors and omissions," negligence and malpractice. (For licensed practitioners.)
3. Product liability protects against suits resulting from consumer injuries using a product you produce. (Custom massage oils, creams, etc.)

Not all liability insurance lines are needed by all practitioners who are sexual healers, it depends on what your healing practice provides. In any case, sexual healers should be conscientious in keeping their healing space free of anything that could inadvertently cause harm to a client by tripping over something, slipping on massage oil, or falling when getting off of the massage table or standing up too fast after being prone for a lengthy period. A healer should make every effort to have a clean space and always use clean sheets and pillowcases including cleaning any surfaces their client's body may touch.

* There are many insurance products that cover liability in different forms, consult an insurance broker or agent for possible products that may apply to your unique services. However, due to the current semi-illicit nature of sexual healing in many localities it may be very difficult to find insurance that will protect you from legal liability.

Currently, it appears that the best things to do to avoid legal liability are:

1. Screen your clients thoroughly with a competent intake process.
2. Provide clients with ample information about your healing practice, the healing process, and what you intend to deliver.
3. Don't over-promise.
4. Do over-deliver—especially ethically.
5. Use attorney reviewed and approved business forms and practices.

There is no protection from criminal liability if law enforcement deems you are acting as a prostitute, pimping, or pandering. In this case, you will likely be prosecuted and will need legal representation. However, I believe it is entirely possible to provide safe sexual healing services without attracting undue or unwanted attention as long as the sexual healer doesn't flaunt community readiness for such a service in their advertising marketing and doesn't inflate and misrepresent their service to the public.

There are ways to present yourself and methods of best business practices that may reduce your exposure to being arrested or sued (See section:s on Informed Consent, Disclosure and Confidentiality, Good Business Practices, and Marketing-Getting Clients). These methods are not advice on how to defy the law, but how to do your best to work within existing legal and regulatory structures with ethical standards. To be clear, until laws change and community standards become more enlightened there are no guarantees—all you can do is try to minimize your exposure.

Disclosure and Confidentiality

Besides *informed consent,* there are other principles that have legal ramifications and requirements that bear on consent and private information and are important for sexual healers and clients to be aware of.

In California and many other states and municipalities, if a practitioner is not licensed it is required by law that they provide a Disclosure Statement that reveals to potential clients the fact that the practitioner is unlicensed. This falls under the "buyer beware" principle as well as acknowledges an adult's right to choose what treatment they receive and with whom they will receive it from in their pursuit of health and wellbeing. Sexual Healers who are not licensed under some other auspices must comply with this legal mandate where it is required by state or local government.

Client-practitioner confidentiality is another legal exposure to be aware of. Not only is it a good ethical practice to not reveal personal information about someone in your care and treatment, but you may also be liable for a civil or statutory suit if you disclose it. There are certain legal exceptions where confidentiality can, or will, be breached (with and without consent) which generally are:

- With written consent, the practitioner may consult with the client's treating physician or another healthcare provider to coordinate care;
- In an emergency; sufficient information may be shared to address an immediate emergency the client is facing;
- If the client poses a threat of harm to their self, to another person, or to the community;
- In the event of psychiatric hospitalization;
- If the client reports information indicating that a child, disabled, or elderly person is suffering abuse or neglect;
- Following a court order, issued by a judge, could require a practitioner to release information about the client's counseling and healing program, or could require the practitioner to testify;

Confidentiality extends beyond disclosing personal information to the public, strangers, institutions or other parties not qualified or approved to receive it. Additional considerations include business communications and circumstances where others may see private information (such as phone messages, emails, or social media posts). In addition, there may be circumstances where sexual healing practitioners encounter clients in social situations; and to be *familiar* with the client might reveal to others accompanying them that they are working with a sexual healer. Consideration of confidential information and the healer-client relationship also includes taking care to not reveal to family members, children, and spouses of clients that a client is working with a sexual healer.

Clergy-Penitent Privilege

Information disclosed to clergy, a pastoral, or spiritual counselor during the course of counseling, advising, or conveying spiritual direction is deemed "privileged communication" and held in the strictest confidence possible under the legal auspices of "clergy-penitent privilege." [38]

In cases where a sexual healer is an ordained minister, there is what's called the *clergy-penitent privilege.* This is a legal mechanism that prevents clergy or spiritual counselors from being required to disclose confidential communications in a court proceeding. This privilege belongs to the person who disclosed the information and is designed for their protection, rather than for the protection of the clergy. In other words, a sexual healer who is an ordained minister can claim clergy-penitent privilege to protect the client but not to protect themselves. If they are accused of abuse or assault clergy-penitent privilege will not help them.

Deepening and Improving a Sexual Healing Practice

The ideal that a sexual healer strives for is to serve their client as an adept and responsible steward of session activities which stay on-track and in-sync with their client's consent and intention to heal. To maintain this ability, sexual healers must expand and deepen their self-knowledge and experience with competently moderating their emotions and behavior, as well as adding to their expertise concerning sexual healing methods and treatments.

In addition, healers should maintain a practice that provides additional and continuing education and experience in areas related to sexual healing like psychology, physiology, and subtle energy systems.

Dual Awareness & Self Control

Dual awareness[39][40] is the ability to observe more than one experience simultaneously. For sexual healers, this includes an objective observation that monitors what is happening and simultaneously, an awareness of the subjective emotion-thought reaction to what is happening. Dual awareness allows a sexual healer to observe the transference-countertransference influences that arise in a session and moderate the impulsive desires/thoughts/emotions and behavior that these prompt.

To cultivate the self-control that dual awareness provides, a sexual healer must be able to consciously separate within their awareness the 'what's so' facts of an experience and the prompted intervening feelings, thoughts, and reactive behavior which arises within the mind—before they are acted upon with words or behavior. One of the best tools for cultivating self-control and dual awareness is meditation.

Meditation Practice

For sexual healers, meditation is useful in accomplishing several objectives:

- Mental and Psychic focus
- Mental/Emotional/Energetic clearing
- Moderating and Conditioning Personal Energy Resonance

Meditation that fosters mental and psychic focus by repeating a mantra or focusing on a symbol or a singular point of focus strengthens the mind's ability to remain aware of the objective and subjective experience in a state of conscious oversight. This type of meditation assists a sexual healer to maintain dual awareness during sessions and be able to make choices that don't allow personal issues, desires or fantasies, to influence a session, nor be influenced by a client's projections.

Meditation that creates mental/emotional clearing by releasing thoughts and emotions as they arise fosters a relaxed and open state of awareness that promotes an objective 'witness' perspective. This is an essential state of awareness that creates conscious oversight which prevents a healer from unconsciously giving into transference-countertransference influences during a session with a client.

During a session, the optimum state of mind and emotion for a sexual healer is to be able to recognize spontaneous intervening desires, thoughts, and behavior prompts that have the potential to take the session off-track or harm the client in some way, and make conscious choices that keep the session within consent boundaries and in line with the client's current state and their ability to absorb and integrate session treatments safely.

Another way that meditation benefits a sexual healer is in its ability to moderate and condition their emotional and energetic resonance to be clear of vibrational 'debris' which can originate with the client's or a healer's personal issues and experiences.

Meditation combined with yogic or Taoist energy clearing and grounding practices is very effective in maintaining the proper personal energy resonance when interacting with clients and in clearing and releasing energetic debris resulting from interacting with clients. This is a type of active meditation that contributes to conscious breath control, which strengthens a healer's ability to be mindfully present and moderate their emotions and maintain objective awareness.

For these reasons and more, meditation is an essential tool for personal and professional development and in maintaining a sexual healing practice which is clear of contaminating elements by either the healer's personal issues or the client's projections of their issues.

Inner Work

The most important thing for a sexual healer to be able to detect and handle is their own personal issues. Inner work is a method of introspection and self-exploration and healing developed by noted psychotherapist C.G. Jung and promoted by his student Robert A. Johnson in his book "Inner Work." (see Reading List appendix)

Sexual healers should be adept at doing their inner work to reveal more about their personal "shadow" aspects, and fantasies and projections. They should know themselves as deeply and pervasively as possible in an ongoing self-revealing endeavor. Not only are there issues and wounds from the past which they must process and integrate, but there will also be ongoing current manifestations of shadow aspects that will arise.

The goal is to become adept at processing one's shadow readily and fluently whenever it manifests to prevent unconsciously projecting or acting-out their shadow with a client. A regular practice of meditative self-inquiry and mindful examination of the thoughts and emotions that come up during sessions which trigger, challenge, or activate a healer's personal shadow will reveal where there is more inner work that can be done.

To assist with this self-evaluation and moderation, sexual healers do well to have post-session reviews to discuss their insights and disclosures with a trusted coach or mentor to process, integrate and release their unconscious reactions or patterns and reveal hidden desires, to be as clear and grounded, and as positively effective as possible when working with clients.

There is always a transference-countertransference going on with a client during sessions. Having deep self-knowledge and self-awareness will help to ensure that this transference-countertransference won't infect a session and possibly cause harm to a client. Healers must be able to recognize and contain their personal desires and moderate their behavior and remain as neutral and objective as possible.

Additional Training

Sexual healing is a unique mixture of addressing a client's emotional, psychological, spiritual, and physiological symptoms stemming from sexual trauma wounds. Treatments address the client's emotional, somatic, energetic, and erotic levels of consciousness integration to encourage symptom release and recovery. It's therefore practical for sexual healers to round out their knowledge and experience in related treatment methods and broaden the areas of their experience and understanding to better serve their clients' needs.

Get additional training or do research on:

- Psychology and Emotion. Understanding what's going on at conscious and unconscious levels of awareness and how the mind processes experiences that overwhelm and wound the psyche.
- Human developmental stages and what happens when emotional-psychological damage occurs.
- Somatic therapy. Understanding the psychological and emotional effects of touch therapy and the development of a healthy mind-body-emotion integration.
- Bioenergetics—the body's energy system—and how trauma, anxiety, stress, and sex are processed and the energetic effects on personal awareness and well-being.
- Complimentary care, or alternative healing methods such as Myofascial Release and Visceral Manipulation that address the nexus of emotion, energy, and physiology.

Maintain a Professional Practice

Sexual healers should strive to be the best possible alternative healthcare facilitator that they can be and to be a positive influence in the greater community of sexual healers. Ideally, they would also establish relationships with professionals in other fields to form informal or formal networks of mutual support and referral.

A sexual healer is rarely the sole resource of healing for their clients. It's good to have a network of other professionals in related fields that healers refer clients to including modalities like energy work, deep tissue massage, Myofascial Release, Emotional Intelligence, Somatic

Experiencing, coaching/counseling/therapy, nutrition and diet, and spiritual guidance.

Sexual Healing Session Do's and Don'ts

Do

- Establish and maintain Consent, and the integrity of the session's container.
- Perform frequent check-ins to make sure of a client's state of consent and ability to handle and absorb their experience.
- When beginning a new treatment or phase of treatments, ask about the client's readiness to proceed, and only proceed at a pace the client is in consent with.
- Present yourself as a professional, wearing clothing that doesn't make a client feel uneasy or overwhelmed.
- Find within yourself, empathy with the client's condition and wounds—someplace where you have had a similar experience and have processed a similar wound.
- Remain present and observant of the client's state of being and reactions to treatments—especially the onset of dissociative states and bring them back to present awareness.
- Be mindful of what is coming up for you during a session and if needed, take breaks to compose yourself or process something.
- Pause or end a session if a client is unable to absorb or contain their experience and maintain conscious awareness and consent with what is happening in the session.

Don't

- Spontaneously or with short notice, change the direction of a session to include treatments that weren't previously discussed and consented to.

- Decide to impulsively test a boundary or introduce an interaction which is beyond a client's consent or ability to handle or assimilate in the moment.
- Have expectations for what a client should be able to handle or tolerate. Meet the client where they are at and work from there.
- Strip naked with a client. Exposing your genitals with a client is likely to activate their sexual trauma and confuse their understanding of the session's intention and consent boundaries.
- Lie on top of a client. Female clients especially can feel assaulted and emotionally harmed—triggering sexual assault memories of being pinned down.
- Project your personal needs onto the client, or feel you are due sexual attention by offering or pressuring the client to have intercourse or engage sexually with you.
- Take advantage of a client's state of somatic trance or Tantric thrall and cross consent boundaries or sexually assault your client.
- Check-out into a personal fantasy with the client.

The Session

The sexual healing session is where everything comes together to address, explore, discover, process, integrate, and release, the issues, and causes of symptoms that impact a survivor of sexual abuse. The session happens in a consciously created container that provides a safe place for healing, transformation, and growth to occur.

It is important that the service being offered to a client and the intent and container of a session's activities and boundaries be clearly defined and understood, with all applied treatments and activities consented with.

Consent Confusion

These days there are more people open to alternative, complementary healing methods, or consciousness expanding experiences led by a spiritual teacher, thought leader, or alternative healer guiding a group or a private healing session into expanded states of mind and somatic experience. These experiences utilize the participant's psychic readiness, openness, and their trust in the facilitator, to evoke emotions, realizations and revelations that affect positive transformation and healing. However, it's also true that this state of openness can put unprepared and vulnerable survivors of sexual abuse in jeopardy of being taken advantage of and harmed.

Some unscrupulous healers or teachers may exploit confusing and vague boundaries and the client's vulnerable emotional state to take advantage of them. The abuse can happen as a kind of "bait and switch" with the client feeling they were at least partly responsible for the harm they experienced because they agreed to participate in the session—feeling like they had to endure the undesired treatment to get to the healing they were seeking.

Case study: A client shared with me her experience with an energy worker who said he would balance her Chakras and do some lymphatic drainage massage, which she agreed to. During the intake discussion, the energy worker revealed that he also offers sexual healing, and if after energy clearing and lymphatic massage it seemed right for the client -and if she signed a release- he could provide that service also.

After some time into the session, while receiving bodywork she had relaxed deeply and drifted into a somatic trance, he began to engage her genitals which made her uncomfortable and tense up. She asked for a break and after coming back from the bathroom, he asked for her consent to continue with the additional level of sexual healing work. She refused the offer and confronted him about crossing boundaries and failing to do what he said was his protocol (obtaining consent and a signed release from her). It was too little consideration, too late for her—she already felt assaulted by his manipulation and crossed boundaries.

She told me, "My right as an autonomous woman to 'stop here' was taken from me." But she also shared that she felt conflicted about feeling co-responsible for her abuse because she had agreed to the session. This example shows how quickly boundaries can be crossed when a client is in a vulnerable state and the healer loses their focus and assumes what a client wants without obtaining consent. Creating and maintaining safety during sexual healing sessions is an ongoing exercise of conscious awareness and perceptive consideration of the consent boundaries which should be repeatedly affirmed between healer and client during the session.

Creating Safety

The sexual healing session is the container in which the client's fears and vulnerabilities are revealed and worked with to enable the client to return to feeling whole and empowered again. Clients have a broad spectrum of fears, including fears of inadequacy and failure, fears about sexual naïveté and performance, and fears about connection, touch, trust, and intimacy.

For many survivors of sexual assault, their healing involves overcoming shame and taking back their personal power and rebuilding their sense of wholeness. Initial sessions can often be about releasing anger, deep emotional pain, and shame which then makes room for nurturing their sensual awareness, and sexual empowerment.

As mentioned previously, the client's process of dealing with their wounds of abuse, assault, or molestation start long before the sexual healing session occurs. They are likely to have trepidation about safety and trust, and it is in the sexual healing session that these concerns will either be relieved or affirmed. It is essential that the sexual healer provides an adequate intake process to not only gather essential information but to also begin to address the client's trepidation and concern for safety and competency.

Pre-session Intake

Each client will have their own symptoms, psychological and emotional issues and wounds they are dealing with. Sexual healers should provide ample opportunity for a client to express themselves and ask questions so they can feel more confident with sexual healing and with the healer.

It's a good practice to use a set of basic questions that will help the sexual healer understand the client's unique condition and the personal issues they are dealing with. Open-ended questions about their state of mind and emotional challenges open the door for more details to follow up on. (See "The Healer: Desires, Fears, and Boundaries" section) In addition, questions about physical condition, alcohol, and prescription or recreational drug use, as well as general living circumstances and current relationship, will inform the work done later in sessions.

Showing genuine warmth, empathy, and understanding during the intake process will help the client open up and feel safe to share the story of their personal wounding and struggle. This is also the time for the healer to assess if the client is or is not a good fit for them as well. There can be various reasons a healer, or a client decides that the potential for working together is not a good fit. Either the healer or the client could simply have a feeling or intuition that they aren't a good match to work together. If a sexual healer decides a potential client is not a good fit to work with, it's appropriate to provide an explanation that helps them understand that it's not a personal rejection.

Some reasons a healer might decide someone is not a good fit to work with:

- The healer may feel the client's symptoms/condition are beyond the healer's experience or knowledge to address,
- The healer may feel the client is not ready for sexual healing treatments and would be better served to work with a therapist before taking on sexual healing,
- The healer might have a personal issue which the client triggers in the healer—throwing them off their balance, groundedness, and objectivity.
- The healer may feel the client is too unbalanced emotionally, or that they are seeing sexual healing as a date or an opportunity for a personal romantic relationship.

Some reasons a client might choose to not work with a particular healer:

- The client doesn't feel safe due to demonstrated behavior of the healer or due to their intuitive hit of the healer's energy.
- The healer doesn't demonstrate sufficient awareness, knowledge, or experience in working with the client's symptoms or condition.
- The client feels there is an energetic mismatch, which is tied to a similar intuitive hit of incompatibility.
- The client feels the healer is "coming onto them,"—flirting and trying to establish a personal romantic relationship.

Under Psychiatric Care?

The scope of intake questions should also inform the sexual healer about the client's previous experience working with other healers or therapists and any medications they may be taking that may affect their ability to absorb and process what is happening during the healing session.

If a client is under the care of a psychiatrist or licensed therapist, it's good to ask the client if their therapist knows about their client's sessions with the sexual healer and to try to work with the client in a way that considers and supports their therapist's treatment.

Other areas for discussion during the pre-session intake should include the client's history with other healers (especially other sexual healers) and their familiarity with esoteric subjects such as the Chakra energy system and working with sexual energy as it is typically taught in Tantra.

Legal Disclaimer, Informed Consent, Disclosure Statements

The intake session is also the appropriate time to present all of the legal and best practices documents about policies and procedures which the client should read carefully and sign before treatment begins in sessions.

Essential Elements of a Session

Intention & Container

To avoid causing harm a sexual healer should co-create with the client a clear intention for the session that accurately represents the client's resolve for the desired transformation. In addition to this, the sexual healer and client should discuss and come to a clear understanding about the session's container in terms of boundaries and behaviors for the session. The sexual healer is responsible for stewarding the session and keeping to the agreement of the session's intention and container.

Consent Discussion

During the process of creating an intention and container, reaching a mutually considered consent is essential. Consent allows the client to participate in the session with full approval and as an empowered co-creator in the healing process. Rather than being something to avoid discussing, informed consent can be a great asset and tool for facilitating healing (see the previous section on Consent).

Frequent Check-ins

Frequently checking in with the client—erring on the side of more, rather than less—confirms consent and informs the healer of what is happening in the client's experience and keeps the container clear and in support of the healing alliance.

To check-in during a session ask simple questions like "what are you feeling?" or "what's happening for you?" or "how are you doing?" After listening and discussing what is revealed, follow up with questions about continuing like "what would you like to do now?" or "are you ready for the next step?" Notice that most of these questions do not have a simple yes or no answer. They invite a descriptive response that will give the sexual healer deeper insight and guidance on what is best for the client. The answer to these questions will inform the healer of how the client is doing emotionally and in feeling if they are keeping within the intention and container of the session.

Ethical Behavior

During a sexual healing session, it is paramount that the healer stays within the boundaries consented to in pre-session discussions. Ethical behavior that supports the client's desire to heal and transcend previous limitations doesn't subvert this intention (by making the session about the sexual healer) but keeps the focus on the client's needs and desire for healing and wholeness.

Ethical behavior also maintains the confidential nature of the professional relationship with a client and respects each client's right to privacy. Ethical sexual healers do not discuss personal details or reveal the identity of their clients in conversations with others.

Most important things to know or ask questions about before a session:

Session Questions for the Healer:

- What is the intention and purpose of the session?
- Do I have to be undressed?
- Are you going to be undressed?
- What treatments or activities will be included?

  o What is their purpose?
  o Is sensual touch used, if so where?
  o Are invasive treatments (vaginal/anal penetration) part of the session? If so, will gloves be worn?

- What will I be doing? What is expected of me?
- What will you be doing?
- How do I signal I'm overwhelmed, I need a break, or I'm "checking out?"
- What are your boundaries and limits—what will NOT be happening?
- What are the likely side effects of session treatments?

Session Questions for the Client:

- What are your top concerns about sexual healing sessions and their treatments?
- What outcome are you seeking from sexual healing treatments?
- What additional support do you have? If needed, is there someone who can be available for you after the session with additional support, and in between sessions?
- What are your fears about me or the session?
- What are your boundaries and limits—what will not be happening?
- Are you on any medications, alcohol, or recreational drugs?

The sexual healing session should be the place where there is complete trust in what is happening or will happen and there is good rapport communication where client and healer easily share observations and feelings about what is happening to ensure the container of consent is accurate and current for the client.

In so doing, the client can relax and open to the session treatments and activities and allow their effects to do their work and facilitate the client's healing. Sexual healers who provide this integrity and steward healing sessions ethically are an invaluable resource for sexual trauma survivors.

A Code of Ethics for Sexual Healers

This Code of Ethics is a summary statement of suggested standards by which sexual healers agree to conduct their practices and is a declaration of principles that foster acceptable, ethical, and professional behavior safeguarding the interests and wellbeing of clients.

A Sexual Healer:

- Maintains a sincere commitment to provide the highest quality care to those who seek their services.
- Performs only those services they are qualified to offer and requested to do as represented by their education, certification, affiliation, experience, and other qualifications.
- Accurately informs their clients of the scope and limitations of their abilities and **obtains the informed and voluntary consent** of the client before providing treatment.
- Respects a client's boundaries and right to choose or deny treatment while keeping the client fully informed of treatment options and possibilities, especially in areas that may challenge a client's experience or trust.
- Acknowledges the confidential nature of the professional relationship with a client and respects each client's right to privacy.
- Strives for personal and professional excellence through regular self-assessment of personal strengths, limitations, and effectiveness, including supplemental continuing education and training.

- Conducts business and professional activities with honesty and integrity.
- Avoids any activity or interaction that might be in conflict with the best interests of the client.

Conclusion

Applying safe sexual healing practices is paramount for a client's protection and wellbeing as well as to support the reputation of sexual healing as a respectable and effective alternative healing modality. Due to the psychological vulnerability and physical intimacy inherent in sexual healing treatments, it is extremely important that sexual healers be well trained and have an adept awareness of their own psychological issues, as well as being acutely attuned to the client's sensitivity, emotional edge, and ability to absorb and process session treatments.

Sexual Healers are responsible for their client's wellbeing during sessions as well as the resulting aftereffects of treatments. Clients are responsible for obtaining sufficient information about a healer's expertise and practices to reach trust and confidence in working with them. Under the guidance of the healer, the client participates in co-creating the consent container of behavior and activity boundaries within a session. Clients and sexual healers are both responsible for supporting the healing alliance and maintaining consent and whole-hearted participation ongoingly during a session. However, it is the healer who bears the greatest responsibility in stewarding sessions with integrity that protects the client from harm. Major shifts in treatment should be discussed thoroughly prior to their enactment and should be applied in a *future* session to allow for ample consideration of consent.

My intention and hope is that this guidebook is an informative resource for the ethical and responsible implementation of sexual healing treatments and methods in sessions for both sexual healers and their clients. It is also my hope that it will help to educate, inform, guide and inspire sexual healers, their potential clients, and the uninformed public, to have confidence in the sexual healing process and be able to participate as empowered co-creators in achieving healing and returning to wholeness.

Appendix

Sexual Healing Training Resources:

American Board of Sexology

americanboardofsexology.com

Institute for Advanced Study of Human Sexuality (IASHS)

www.humansexualityeducation.com

The American College of Sexologists International

www.americancollegeofsexologists.org

Sexological Bodywork

www.sexologicalbodywork.com

Association of Certified Sexological Bodyworkers

sexologicalbodyworkers.org

Institute of Somatic Sexology

instituteofsomaticsexology.com

Sexological Bodywork Training UK

sexologicalbodywork.co.uk

Reading List

Psychology

Johnson, Robert A. (1986). *Inner Work: using dreams & active imagination for personal growth.*

Neumann, Erich (1962). *The Origins and History of Consciousness Part II: the psychological states in the development of personality.*

Edinger, Edward F. (1972). *Ego and Archetype.*

Von Franz, Marie-Lousie (1999). *Archetypal Dimensions of the Psyche.*

Washburn, Michael (2003). *Embodied Spirituality in a Sacred World.*

Qualls-Corbett, Nancy (1988). *The Sacred Prostitute: Eternal Aspect of the Feminine.*

Sedgwick, D. (1994). *The wounded healer: countertransference from a Jungian perspective.*

McNeely, Deldon Anne (1987). *Touching: body therapy and depth psychology.*

Ford, Debbie (1998). *The Dark Side of the Light Chasers: Reclaiming your power, creativity, brilliance, and dreams.*

Ford, Debbie (2002). *The Secret of the Shadow: the power of owning your whole story.*

Relationship and Communication

Rosenberg, Marshall B. (1999). *Nonviolent Communication: a language of compassion.*

Schnarch, David (2009). *Intimacy & Desire: Awaken the passion in your relationship.*

Sanford, John A. (1980). *The Invisible Partners: how the male and female in each of us affects our relationships.*

The Body's Energy System

Lowen, Alexander (1975, 1983). *Bioenergetics: the revolutionary therapy that uses the language of the body to heal the problems of the mind.*

Lowen, Alexander (1988). *Love, Sex, and Your Heart: the health-happiness connection.*

Rosenberg, Jack Lee (1985). *Body, Self, & Soul: Sustaining integration.*

Myss, Caroline (1996). *Anatomy of the Spirit: the seven stages of power and healing.*

Smith, Fritz Frederick (1998). *Inner Bridges: a guide to energy movement and body structure.*

Angelo, Jack (1997). *Hands-On Healing: a practical guide to channeling your healing energies.*

Andrews, Ted (1993). *The Healer's Manual: a beginner's guide to vibrational therapies.*

Gordon, Richard (1999). *Quantum-Touch: the power to heal.*

Trauma Healing

Rothschild, Babette. (2000). *The Body Remembers.*

Levine, Peter A. (1997). *Waking the Tiger: Healing Trauma*

Van der Kolk, Bessel M.D. (2015). *The Body Keeps the Score: Brain, Mind, and Body in the Healing of Trauma*

Endnotes

1 http://en.wikipedia.org/wiki/Ahimsa
2 Britton, Patti O. (2005). The art of sex coaching: expanding your practice.
3 http://www.jungny.com/lexicon.jungian.therapy.analysis/carl.jung.157.html
4 Lowen, A. (1975 p. 14,15). Bioenergetics. New York: Coward, McCann & Geoghegan.
5 Ibid (p. 92)
6 Ibid (p. 93)
7 https://traumahealing.org/about-us/
8 https://www.sciencedaily.com/terms/oxytocin.htm
9 http://theutopianlife.com/2014/10/14/hacking-into-your-happy-chemicals-dopamine-serotonin-endorphins-oxytocin/
10 https://www.merriam-webster.com/dictionary/consent
11 http://en.wikipedia.org/wiki/Informed_consent
12 https://1in6.org/the-1-in-6-statistic/
13 http://www.oneinfourusa.org/statistics.php
14 http://www.victimsofcrime.org/media/reporting-on-child-sexual-abuse/child-sexual-abuse-statistics
15 https://www.ncjrs.gov/pdffiles1/nij/183781.pdf
16 https://gurumag.com/tantric-abuse-articles/
17 http://apps.who.int/classifications/icd10/browse/2010/en#/F43.0
18 http://psychcentral.com/disorders/acute-stress-disorder-symptoms/
19 http://en.wikipedia.org/wiki/Acute_stress_reaction
20 Sedgwick, D. (1994). The wounded healer: countertransference from a Jungian perspective. London: Routledge. (pg. 1)
21 http://www.bendpsychology.com/Articles/Transference.htm
22 Sedgwick, D. (1994). The wounded healer: countertransference from a Jungian perspective. London: Routledge. (pgs. 105-109)
23 Ibid (pg. 12)
24 https://www.cdc.gov/std/hpv/stdfact-hpv.htm
25 Qualls-Corbett, N. (1988). The sacred prostitute: eternal aspect of the feminine.
26 Shepsut, Asia (1993). Journey of the Priestess: the Priestess Traditions of the Ancient World, a Journey of Spiritual Awakening and Empowerment

27 http://en.wikipedia.org/wiki/Epic_of_Gilgamesh

28 Schärf Kluger, Rivkah (1991). *The Archetypal Significance of Gilgamesh: A Modern Ancient Hero* (pgs. 32–51)

29 http://en.wikipedia.org/wiki/Transubstantiation

30 https://www.dictionary.com/browse/ego

31 McNeely, D. A. (1987). *Touching: body therapy and depth psychology.* Toronto: Inner City Books

32 http://en.wikipedia.org/wiki/Energy_%28esotericism%29

33 http://therapists.psychologytoday.com/rms/content/therapy_methods.html

34 http://blogs.psychcentral.com/therapy-soup/2011/01/therapy-tools-role-playing/

35 http://definitions.uslegal.com/p/pandering/

36 http://definitions.uslegal.com/p/prostitution/

37 http://dictionary.law.com/Default.aspx?selected=1151

38 https://www.hg.org/legal-articles/application-and-limitations-of-the-clergy-privilege-40305

39 Rothschild, B. (2000). *The Body Remembers.* (pp 132–135)

40 https://www.synergiacounselling.com/using-dual-awareness-to-deal-with-traumatic-memoriesemotional-flashbacks/

Index

Printed in the United States
By Bookmasters